Keep on Moving!

By Coach Tregs

(Founder of 30 Plus Men's Fitness)

Dedication

I would like to dedicate this book to my late, great friend Mark Ramskill.

Thank you for your support and encouragement in the early days.

Although we only knew each other for three years before you passed away, your belief in me gave me the confidence to never give up on our vision.

Keep on Truckin' brother!

Acknowledgements

I WOULD LIKE TO ACKNOWLEDGE both my mum and dad who showed me how to live an active life from a very young age.

Some of my earliest memories (around eight or nine years old) are of running around the block back home in Gloucester with my mum, or kicking a ball about with my dad in a local park.

Several years later, I stood at the back of my mum's aerobics classes, watching with pride as she led thirty or forty ladies with energy and confidence.

Meanwhile, dad was actively involved with my football set-up; picking me and my mates up and driving us home and helping out with the coaching too.

In my teens, my mum drove me around the South West (with a bike rack on the car) to enable me to compete in Mountain bike events. My dad did the same and watched me compete in multiple Cross-Country events for years.

Thank you to Sarah, my amazing partner and

mother of our two boys John and Elliot. Thank you for putting up with me working all hours in pursuit of my dream; for keeping me grounded when I get crazy ideas and for being the practical and sensible one in our relationship!

Finally, to my two sons John and Elliot who are the apple of my eye and who are growing into two fine young boys. It makes me proud to see you brimming with energy, confidence and a zest for getting outdoors.

Words can never express how much I love you and how much your spur me on to become a better person daily.

You are both the present and the future and I am so grateful for your continued health and happiness.

I love being on this journey called life with you both.

About the Author

Mark Tregilgas (Coach Tregs) currently resides at his home in the Vale of Glamorgan, South Wales with his partner Sarah, his dad, two sons and two dogs.

His passion and love for his work continues today through one-to-one private coaching in Cardiff, his Bootcamp and his online business. He is also head coach and assistant coach with his sons Under 8 and Under 10 football teams respectively. When he is not working online or training clients, he dedicates his time to coaching kids and organising teams for matches each weekend.

#30plusmensfitness
Facebook: 30 Plus Mens Fitness
Instagram: @30plusmensfitness
Website: www.30plusmensfitness.com
https://5daybusydadtransformationchallenge.com/

Table of Contents

CHAPTER ONE

Introduction

ON MONDAY 22nd MARCH 2021, we reached the first anniversary of the Coronavirus lockdown. At the same time, around 18,000 words in, I shelved this book. I had been training hard for the Manchester Marathon and had just started my taper.

Then came the national lockdown.

Not only was the marathon itself cancelled, gyms were closed as well as all outdoor training. We were told to stay at home.

This meant I had to stop training clients, both in and out of the gym. It's fair to say that my head was fried and I was fearful for the future.

Returning to finish this book was the last thing on my mind at the outset of the national emergency.

Today, one year on, I cannot explain how grateful I am for lockdown. It gave me the opportunity to level up – not just my online activities, but also my physical fitness and mind-set.

If you are a new client reading this, it's highly likely you became part of my '30 Plus' online world during that first lockdown of 2020. Perhaps you are a client from before lockdown. Either way, anyone who is part of my 30-Plus Men's Fitness community knows that it was the beginning of lockdown that things began to change massively for me.

I didn't know it at the time, but as I write this today, I can wholeheartedly tell you that during the last 12 months, I experienced an incredible 'shift'.

The shift – physical, mental and spiritual – means that I believe I can offer you more knowledge in this book than I could have ever done pre-pandemic.

In March 2020 I weighed around 90kgs. To-day, one year on, I'm almost 10kgs lighter. I haven't touched alcohol for almost nine months, and my fitness levels have gone through the roof. Physically, I'm in the best shape of my life – at the age of forty-two.

I have changed my thought processes, training

regime, recovery process and eating habits. These changes mean that I can deliver more to you from the things I've learned. Throughout this narrative, I will refer to experiences, not just during the previous twelve months, but also from my earlier years. I will show you what you can learn from them.

I am enormously excited to be able to help you on this journey – the road to health, fitness and contentment.

So, let's get started…

CHAPTER TWO

Dedication – Mark Ramskill

I CANNOT BEGIN THIS BOOK without dedicating it to my late, great friend, Mark Ramskill. Mark sadly passed away in 2012 after taking his own life.

I met Mark back in 2009 when he came to me as a personal training client. Even though I only knew Mark for three years in total, he made more of an impact on me than any other person in my life (excluding my partner or family, of course).

I truly believe I was meant to meet him and that the universe brought us together at just the right time.

I vividly remember the first day he came to train with me. I peered out of the gym window and saw this tall, gangly fella pacing around the car park. He looked nervous as hell. When he arrived at the door, his face was stricken with anxiety, but after just one session, we had really hit it off.

Mark was not from around here, but he had moved to Cardiff for work. Like myself, I had moved from Gloucestershire to Cardiff for University. The fact that we had many things in common, meant that we hit it off immediately. We were both Englishmen, we liked similar music and we had a similar sense of humour. Mark loved old-school hip-hop which was a sound I had grown up on. Our banter was the same, though quite twisted at times!

Mark hated exercise and told me that any cardio exercise had to be off-limits. However, he fell in love with weight training. Some of my fondest memories are of us lifting tin with some 'Ice Cube' or 'Ole dirty Bastard' blasting.

Sometimes we would train together after the gym had officially closed. It was just the two of us, which meant we could blare music as loud as we wanted and share 'close to the bone' banter without anyone overhearing!

He would turn up with this huge old-school ghetto blaster and we would play the most explicit hip-hop whilst screaming at each other doing weights. It was fucking brilliant.

He told me that he had never enjoyed any type of training before, but he was really getting into the weights. I'd see him a few times a week and our friendship grew quickly.

Mark worked in digital media. I had no idea what that was and never really gave it too much thought. However, when I came up with the idea of '30 Plus Boot camp' in 2010, Mark was the first person I told.

I'd been following bloggers and fitness professionals in the States who were talking about training groups and selecting your perfect niche market. I knew Mark could help. His response was so encouraging.

"I love it mate, and I can help bring it to life. I can record some content for you. I'll help you to set up a YouTube channel and grow a Facebook page."

This was just what I needed. All of that stuff was pretty alien to me. Back in 2010, there weren't many fitness professionals using those platforms.

Mark did exactly what he promised and helped me bring '30 Plus Boot camp' to life.

He attended the first ever session back in May 2010 and, whilst he didn't join in, he filmed loads of action, which can still be found on YouTube. We were up and running!

I stopped charging Mark for personal training

in return for his digital media skills. Under his guidance, we created new content regularly. I had no idea how this content would serve me, but this was Mark's area of expertise and I allowed him to guide me.

I ended up moving into the same apartment block as Mark. Some of my original YouTube content was shot on the grounds of the Cardiff Bay residence where we filmed at the weekend.

He told me to think beyond Cardiff. He said that by creating video content, we could take the 30+ message to the world!

"Think of workouts, meal ideas, health advice; all the tips you've given me. And then just put it on camera," he advised.

In the beginning, we must have done multiple takes. I was either talking too fast, tripping over my words or laughing my head off, but we always got there in the end.

Over a mid-week beer, he would say to me: "I'm telling you Tregs, you've got what it takes. You're enthusiastic and likeable. You can motivate people. Just be yourself in front of the camera. This will appeal to the masses."

He fired me up and made me believe in myself. He showed me that the world could be my oyster if I continued to show up online.

We mapped out a vision for online products and a members' area. The plan was to build it so that Mark could eventually leave his job and work full time for '30 Plus Men's Fitness'.

We created content solidly between May 2010 and January 2012. During that time, I hired a business coach. He recommended that we keep '30 Plus Boot camp' for Cardiff only, and use '30 Plus Men's Fitness' online. Mark set up a new website and we were off!

During that time, I also signed up for a very expensive course. It was in Thailand with a fitness professional called Dax Moy. The ten-day course was designed to help you sell products online. It also offered the time, space and solitude to help you build your product.

Mark and I decided it was our next step. We were already creating an online presence and getting the brand out there. In mid-2011, I invested a huge chunk of money to go on the course. Prior to attending, I had to pay it off in installments over a ten-month period.

Having a business coach was already paying off and we were convinced this would take us to the next level. However, something happened prior to going.

People often hear me say "K.O.T." when I sign off on social media. This stands for "Keep on Trucking". I'll tell you why I use this phrase.

Back in August 2010, just four months after launching '30 Plus Boot camp', I was living in the same apartment block as Mark. I'd taken out a twelve-month rental on an apartment. It was for myself and my partner, who I'd been seeing for around eighteen months. She was coming from overseas to join me.

Unfortunately, the relationship ended within just two weeks of us living together. She moved back home and I was heartbroken.

After she moved out, I told my close friends and family what had happened. Returning home to my apartment after an extremely stressful and upsetting day, Mark was there waiting for me. The first thing he did was give me a big hug. I'll never forget it because Mark wasn't the type of bloke to show his feelings. In fact, if he ever saw men hugging, he would have totally taken the piss. However, there he was, giving me a huge man-hug in the hall of our apartment block.

I'd known the guy for only a short time, yet he was there for me at my lowest ebb. We went for a pint and a curry and as I was sat there, crying into my beer, I looked at him and said: "Mate, what am I going to do?"

He looked me straight in the eyes and said "Do what you do best. Get back in the gym, train your clients and keep on truckin'."

I remember it vividly because it was so fucking simple and yet so profound.

That's exactly what I did. Around nine months later, I met my partner Sarah and moved in with her.

When the time came to go to Thailand in March 2012, things were changing for both Mark and me. Sarah was already pregnant with our first son John. Mark had decided to move to York to live with his girlfriend. He said he would still be helping me with the online side of things, but things felt a little different between us. We organized a send-off for him with the boot camp lads but strangely, he never showed.

Either way, I was now about to fly half way across the world to a course in Thailand with one of the UK's finest experts. Not only that, but I was leaving my pregnant partner behind. It was still very early in our relationship and day of all days; it was her birthday! The pressure was really on.

After spending a day travelling, arriving at the luxury villa and meeting the other fitness professionals, we got to work.

We were told we would have to put in some serious hours if we wanted to create our product in ten days. They encouraged us NOT to go out drinking in the evening if we wanted to be productive. I was tired and jet-lagged, but up for the challenge.

However, on the first night, I had a number of missed calls from one of my clients, Robbo. He was one of the guys that Mark had introduced me to at Boot camp.

This was odd as Robbo knew I was away. He kept calling so I texted him back. Robbo insisted I pick up. He said it was about Mark.

I knew it must be serious.

Robbo broke the news. Mark had passed away.

He had taken his own life following an argument with his partner.

I knew that Mark suffered with anxiety and depression – it was one of the reasons he started training with me. I also knew he had a 'darker side', but he had never really opened up to me about it.

I guess the darkness had gotten the better of him.

Shocked, I couldn't get my head around what had just happened.

Not only that, but I was halfway across the world with a bunch of people I barely knew, miles away from my pregnant partner, and on a course I had invested a ton of money on.

My head was fried.

I broke the news to my fellow fit pros who all offered support, but I told them I needed time on my own.

I rang my partner immediately as I wasn't sure if I should come home or not. Despite being traumatized, we decided that I should stay on. Mark would have wanted me to make the most of the course since it was such a huge investment.

Devastated, I stayed in my room and finally managed to get some sleep. I must have slept for over twelve hours and when I awoke, my head felt a little clearer. I made myself put on my trainers and go for a run.

As I was running along the beach in Thailand, the heavens opened and lightning lit up the sky. I was caught in a crazy thunder storm. All I had on was a pair of shorts and trainers. I was completely drenched, but somehow, it felt euphoric.

It might sound crazy, but I took it as a sign from the universe. I needed to stay on and finish the course.

The lads back home at Boot camp were already organizing a special send off after Mark's funeral, but I had to try to switch off from social media. I needed to focus on why I was in Thailand.

For the next eight or nine days, for the first time ever and without Mark's guidance, I filmed content alone. Setting up a tripod and camera, I must have recorded sixteen basic bodyweight workouts.

It was challenging. Not only did it feel strange without Mark, but the weather was a mix of thirty-degrees blazing sunshine, combined with humidity and torrential storms.

If you have completed one of my online plans, you will have come across these videos. Now you know the story behind them!

Whilst I managed to record all of my workouts out in Thailand, I didn't finish building my programme. I came home and attended Mark's funeral in York, which was pretty horrific.

His poor partner was distraught and blamed

herself. His suicide came just thirty minutes after their argument. He had also talked about suicide a few weeks before, but she had talked him out of it.

It was a terrible blow. I couldn't help but wonder, if he had reached out to me or the lads, would we have been able to help him?

For several months following Mark's death, I stopped creating content. I didn't record any videos and wrote zero content. I didn't even send a single email to my growing subscribers list that Mark had helped to set up.

I felt completely lost without him. I wondered If I would ever be able to take my methods online. Mixed in with this, I was also in the process of moving to a new home with my partner as we prepared for the birth of our first son.

One day, I was sitting in my office at our new home and I went online to check on the website that Mark had created. Despite not creating anything new in months, I would often check in on the website and watch the videos. They reminded me of my time with Mark.

To my shock and horror, the website and all of its content, had gone.

I tried to refresh the browser multiple times, but it seemed that www.30plusmensfitness.com was no more. Over 2 years of content had gone. I started to panic.

I had to contact the hosting company. It turned out that our bills hadn't been paid, so they were taking the page down.

Normally, they give you two weeks grace before deleting your content. At present, the site was just down; I had a matter of days to save it before everything would be deleted forever.

"No worries!" I exclaimed. "I'll settle the account now and get up-to-date."

The problem however, was bigger than that.

They had never heard of me and the website was owned by a "Mr Mark Ramskill".

As part of our arrangement, Mark had paid for hosting our online content and in return, I had stopped charging him for personal training.

Now, months after his death, and with a stack of unpaid bills, all of our content was about to go.

I tried to explain what had happened; that I was Mark's colleague and he had passed away, but they were adamant they weren't going to give me access.

The only way I would be able to take back the

site was if a member of Mark's family contacted them to confirm the handover.

I sat there in my office contemplating my dilemma. Did I really want to have to ask one of Mark's grieving family members to contact the hosting company?

I seriously thought about just binning it all off. I told myself I had a good personal training business and a successful Boot camp; that was enough. If anyone ever asked what happened to '30-Plus Men's Fitness', I would simply tell them my business partner passed away and I wasn't brave enough to carry on without his guidance.

This was a good enough excuse, right?

However, as I mulled it over, I just had this burning feeling inside of me. I knew I had to sort it out and bring '30-Plus Men's Fitness' to life again.

I remembered the conversations we had. Mark had told me how much he believed in me; in my passion and enthusiasm. He told me I could impact others on a global level online.

I then remembered the time when I was crying into my pint after a shitty break up. He looked me in the eye and told me to 'keep on truckin'. That was all the fire I needed.

I contacted Mark's brother. I had met him at the funeral and we'd had a great chat. I politely asked if he could contact the website hosting company on Mark's behalf.

He was fantastic about it and did everything immediately. The site, and all the content, was back up in days.

A short time later, I sent an email to my list of subscribers. It was the first in what felt like forever. I explained why I hadn't been creating content; that I had been struggling with Mark's death.

Normally when you send these emails, you hit 'send' and don't expect a response. In fact, I don't think I had ever received a response in the short time I'd been sending out emails.

This time, I got a response. It said: "Don't give up, you do make a difference." The person who replied probably can't even remember writing it, but it filled me with such a desire to push on and 'keep on truckin'.

By the close of 2012, and with the help of a guy called Karl Warren, I had launched my first ever online paid programme. Just before his death, Mark had found Karl, a fantastic bloke who helped with graphic design.

Those sixteen bodyweight workouts, filmed in tropical heat and thunder in Thailand whilst grieving my friend's loss, were all worth it.

By May 2013, I was up and running online and had set up my Members' club (now the Brotherhood). The rest, as they say, is history.

I am eternally grateful to Mark. His belief in me helped me to push on and see out our vision. I always rely on those famous words 'Keep on Truckin' when times get tough along the way.

I had a choice that day: call time on '30-Plus Men's Fitness', or keep on truckin'.

I'm so glad I kept on truckin'.

Mark, this book is dedicated to you.

CHAPTER THREE

Why should you listen to me?

THE TITLE OF THIS CHAPTER may sound a bit strange. If you've bought my book, you probably already half trust me. However, I want to clarify why I believe you should listen to me and how I've had success helping so many guys just like you.

Plain and simple, I believe many can relate to me because I've never been one of those ripped personal trainers.

Honestly, I've never been ripped!

However, as I write this, at the age of forty-two, I am hands-down in the best shape of my life. It's all down to the lifestyle I lead – a lifestyle I will teach you about in this book.

If you have followed me for a while, you will know about my struggles, before and during my time as a personal trainer.

I've been out of shape for large parts of my

life, probably more than I've been in shape.

I've been out of shape as a personal trainer. I've been in an okay shape. I've been in horrific shape. Now I'm in a shape I feel happy with.

The struggle is real and I truly believe it's formed a massive part of my journey.

This is what gives me so much empathy for other men struggling. I have battled hard for most of my life and I know just how painful it is.

I've had major battles with food. I bloody love my food, yet at times my relationship with it has been awful.

I've always given 100% with exercise, even when I was clueless as to what I was meant to be doing.

I've said this time and time again: I've got terrible genetics and I'm not afraid to admit it. And yet, it's formed my struggle which in turn has made me commit harder.

I was always the guy that trained fucking loads, but never got the results!

I've never really been able to build huge amounts of muscle or get particularly strong. I went through a phase where this bothered me a lot. You've only got to take a look at my skinny calves (the butt of the joke from all the lads) to see that.

I read a study that said you can tell by a man's ability to build muscle just by looking at their calves! The more muscular the calf, the greater the ability to build muscle over all. Well, that's me fucked then!

Back in 2016, I spent a year hammering them, but with little difference. I've met many men over the years that rock up to boot camp with huge calves. When I ask if they've trained them, they reply 'never'! Life's a bitch, eh?

I've always struggled with building muscle and getting that lean look, yet I've never struggled with the long distance, cardiovascular stuff. The journey that has led me on will hopefully give you many insights and value.

Despite my poor genetics, as I write this, one year into lockdown, I'm 10kgs down in weight in one year. I'm over two hundred days booze-free. I've been tracking pretty much every calorie and gram of protein throughout that time. I can tell you that I'm probably the most comfortable I have ever been with my appearance.

This is simply down to playing the 'long game' that I will evangelize about in this book. This is not to impress you, rather it is to impress upon you, that I know what it's like to struggle.

I understand what it's like to be fat. I first got fat at the age of ten or eleven. I've been fat on and off for many, many years since.

I understand how painful it is to be fat as a kid.

I also understand how painful it is to be fat as an adult.

I understand what it's like to go on holiday, take off your top and hate yourself.

I've suffered with self-hatred at times.

I've cried myself to sleep due to my appearance.

I've started and stopped again more times than I can remember.

I've looked in the mirror and hated my reflection.

I've often been on a holiday with a girlfriend and thought to myself: 'What is she doing with me? I'm a fat mess!'

God knows I've fucking tried! I've tried my hardest; I've trained harder than most, but without any understanding or direction.

I know what it's like not to be able to wear clothes you feel comfortable in.

I know what it's like to wake up after a massive binge on junk food and alcohol, feeling groggy and worthless.

I know what it's like to avoid social occasions because you don't want to be judged about your appearance.

I know what it's like to be a fat personal trainer (the ultimate feeling of failure) because you can't stick to the message you're promoting.

All this really hurts and I expect you are nodding along with me. You might understand when I tell you that I put a brave face on with my bubbly personality, yet inside it was killing me.

So, if you're picking this book up because you're struggling and think you can't ever turn it around, then I know exactly how you're feeling.

I think the heaviest I've been (bear in mind, I'm 5ft 10) is over sixteen stone. You might think that's not heavy, but it's heavy for me!

It's heavy for me – a guy with no calves who holds fat around his belly and chest. Awful genetics and an odd body shape, eh!

It could have been so easy to just say: 'Oh fuck it! I can't build muscle, I can't get in shape, I give up!'

However, I firmly believe these shortcomings are what have driven me on!

I've failed so many times and tried so many

different ways, but it's led me to this stage now.

At the age of forty-two, I feel absolutely amazing; to the point where I feel confident enough to write this book.

I know, hand-on-heart, that it will not only change your life, but prolong it – as long as you follow what I tell you.

It all comes down to lifestyle and not chasing the quick fix. It's about upgrading your mindset. You need to manage your training and nutrition; to build habits that you can maintain for life.

I want you to read this book, understanding that you will never have to 'balls out' again. You will want to make this a lifestyle.

I'll tell you this now; it takes time and it takes patience. It's about the long game.

However, when you crack this, it feels amazing. You'll feel confident because it's both doable and enjoyable. This is quite simply where the magic happens.

I don't care where you are now. You are where you are. I want you to understand that I know how you feel. I simply will not let this fucking consume you for the rest of your life.

If I can fix myself, I can show you how to fix yourself.

I'll show you, step by step, but it's down to you to do the work. It's going to be more enjoyable that you think!

CHAPTER FOUR

Who is this book for?

THERE ARE A WIDE RANGE OF MEN (and women) who follow me; all a variety of shapes and sizes, all with differing levels of fitness.

No matter what shape you are currently in, I simply want to help you improve your life.

You may be that guy who is already very active. Exercise might already play a big part in your life. You may have thought about pushing yourself even further, but you procrastinate about signing up for a challenging event, thinking it's beyond you.

This is your sign: stop procrastinating and sign up for it!

With the help and guidance in this book, I'll make you realise that the only obstacle standing in the way is: You!

However, you might be that guy who is six or stone overweight. You might be thinking: "I slowed down ages ago, what is this book going to do for me?"

This book is going to help you get off the couch and to take those first, critical steps towards losing weight and improving your health.

Wherever you are on your journey, I want this book to light a fire within you to become a better version of yourself.

I am also going to show you a step-by-step improvement process so that by the time you've read this book, you are not only fired up, but have a system to follow. These are systems that I have tested and will explain in detail. Combined with my personal experiences, I will show you how to set up your own system to win.

Whether you want to do Europe's Toughest Mudder or simply be able to climb the stairs without feeling like you're having a cardiac arrest, I promise you will take something from this book.

This book is going to show you that there is no wagon; there is no need to be all-or-nothing. The absolute key is lifestyle.

I cannot re-iterate enough; age should not be a limiting factor. I don't care what you've done in the past; how many times you stopped and started, how many times you've tried new things and failed. This book is going to end all that confusion and all that misery.

Simply read this book, digest it and then put the systems into play.

It's going to change the trajectory of your life with regards to health, fitness and mind-set.

I don't want you to slow down. I'm going to show you how to keep moving forward.

CHAPTER FIVE

Facing your fears and saying 'Fuck it!'

OVER THE YEARS, many people have asked me how I came up with the idea of setting up '30 Plus Men's Fitness'.

I feel it's therefore a great place to start, as many of you won't know my journey prior to being in the fitness industry.

So many people go through life scared to change career, playing it safe and settling for mediocrity because they are so fearful of the unknown.

I'm so glad I faced my fears and changed my career at twenty-six years old. Getting into the fitness industry not only saved my life, but also changed my trajectory forever. It wasn't however, without one of the biggest personal battles. I had to overcome the voices inside telling me I simply 'wasn't good enough'.

In the year 2000, I graduated from the University of Glamorgan in South Wales with a degree in English, Theatre and Media. By then, I was already involved in promoting nightclub events and festivals. Between the ages of nineteen to twenty-four, I was involved in some pretty heavy-duty events. Let's just say, I saw a lot!

I was always a musical man from a young age. I loved house and garage music. Whilst I enjoyed some experiences during this period of my life, not all of them were pleasurable. The nightclub promotion lifestyle was very much a young man's game and extremely risky. One month you would make big and the next, you could lose it all.

I won't lie, I enjoyed the status and perks that came with it. I partied hard. However, at the age of twenty-four, the scene was changing and I was ready to get out.

Being a promoter was often very overwhelming. Your phone would never stop and every Tom, Dick and Harry wanted a freebie.

I got out of the game completely, sold my car, bought a van and became a self-employed courier. Funnily enough, it was a local DJ in the music scene who was also working as a courier, that got me the job.

This was a completely different way of life!

I went from – driving a nice little motor, being the boy-about-town, promoting events and being popular – to delivering parcels in a white van, using a phone that no longer ran off the hook.

The change didn't bother me too much, it was more my friends that were curious. Why would I want to move away from the glamour of the event industry? Why would I want to deliver parcels around the Valleys in a beaten-up old van?

I've always been a grafter and the hours were long, but it didn't bother me. For the first year, I actually enjoyed the peace and quiet of being on my own. No-one was bothering me, threatening me or looking for a guest pass on a Saturday night.

I'd load up my van and drive up the A470 each day listening to Talk Sport and just getting on with it. However, after about a year of that, I started to get twitchy and restless. I began to do some proper soul searching.

When the weather changed into the winter months, it was miserable up in the Valleys: bloody freezing and quite lonely too. I was asking myself a LOT of questions about what I wanted to do with my life.

It also didn't help when friends kept asking: "Tregs, are you going to do this forever? You can do so much more mate. You've got a degree and a big personality. You used to be a promoter. Are you really going to settle for this?"

It hurt me because deep down, I knew they were right. I could offer more, but I just didn't know where to turn.

Driving along in my van, I started to listen to a Spanish language course on CD. I even went back to night school once a week. I decided to learn the language since I had enjoyed so many nice holidays in Spain over the years. I wanted to try something new.

Listening along in the van was great and it kept me very engaged for a while.

After about six months of learning the language, I mentioned to my partner at the time that I would like us to move to Spain. I thought perhaps we could go there and start a new life. We could get work in a bar or something? I was just yearning for change.

She was a Cardiff girl, very close to her family and really wasn't keen on the idea. So, I kept these deep moments of introspection to myself, alone in my van.

I started to go through some pretty big battles with anxiety and depression around that time, which only made matters worse.

I was about twenty-six and my partner was a similar age. We had a nice apartment in Cardiff city centre, but I just had this overwhelming fear of the future. There was a recurring deep concern about turning thirty and not having any direction in life.

Around that time, I struck up a friendship with a guy called Ralph. It worked at one of the businesses I collected mail from. He was about fifteen years older than me and he would say things like: "Tregs you're a great guy! Honestly, don't waste your life – go travelling, see the world!"

He had obviously seen something in me – a spark, a passion. He was only trying to help me, but it added to the worry I was already having about life, work and future.

One day, during one of our frequent conversations, he came out with: "Hey! I've been thinking about becoming a personal trainer."

Even though I wasn't in the fitness industry at

the time, Ralph knew I enjoyed running and was pretty active. He was the same. In fact, I think we may have even met up for a run one day as mates.

He just said he fancied doing something different. He said he'd be able to study for the course whilst sitting on his arse all day at his current job.

That was it: a tiny five-minute conversation before we went on chatting about something else, but it planted a seed in my mind.

A couple of weeks later, Ralph told me about a 10k race happening in Bute Park in Cardiff. The date was February 2006 and the race was the Valentines Love Run. He asked me if I fancied going along. The thing is, despite going for runs to try to lose weight, I hadn't competed a proper distance race for over ten years.

I wasn't in the best of shape, but I thought: 'Fuck it, what the hell!' I fancied a crack at it.

The night before the run, I got a message from Ralph saying that he was unwell and was pulling out of the race. So, I turned up the next day on my own, not really knowing what to expect. I was carrying too much weight, wearing an England FC shell top and footy shorts. My Nike Turtle toe trainers had barely any cushioning or laces!

Most of the other guys were serious runners in all the right gear. I must have stood out like a right thorn!

The race started and off we trotted. As always, I started to get lower back pain, not to mention feelings of tightness in my hamstrings and calves. That always came with carrying too much weight. I also wouldn't have known a mobility routine if it had punched me in the face!

For the first fifteen to twenty minutes, I wasn't really enjoying it, but after a few KM's, I started to loosen up.

I've always had a decent engine, which I'll explain about later in this book. I was starting to feel a bit looser, picking up my pace and moving through.

Some of these runners were eight stone dripping wet, but fifteen-stone fat-boy Tregsy started to overtake them. My confidence began to grow.

Then boom!

Around 5k-6k in, on my second lap, it hit me right in the face; the eureka moment that was to change my life forever. Despite it being mid-February and a tad nippy, it was actually a beautiful morning and the sun was shining. I was now moving through the gears and feeling great.

I was looking up at the sunlight, lost in my thoughts and feeling good. The endorphins were kicking in. I was thinking how awesome it was to be doing something like this on a Saturday morning rather than lying in bed with a hangover.

And then it just hit me.

I'm going to be a personal trainer.

I was twenty-six years old, on the chubby side and trying to lose weight, but always active. I'd been battling anxiety and depression too, but in that moment, none of it mattered. I was having an awakening. It didn't matter where I was in my life currently. This was a calling and everything was going to be okay.

Out of the six hundred runners, I finished the race in the top one hundred that day. That didn't matter – what mattered was that my mind was clear. I knew what I wanted for my future.

I raced home to tell my partner at the time. She had been wonderful, putting up with my anxiety, depression and feelings of being lost. The relief on her face was amazing.

That very afternoon I went straight onto Google and found a personal training course based in Bristol. It was a company called 'Lifetime Health and Fitness'. I couldn't afford to pay for a personal training diploma outright, but I found out I could pay in installments.

Within a few days, I had paid the deposit and I was booked on.

I remember telling close friends that I had decided to become a PT. The initial reaction was quite negative.

"Oh Tregs, I'll say this with love, but you're not really in the best of shape to become a PT, are you?"

"A mate of mine who is ripped tried that and found it really hard to make it work financially."

Some of these comments were coming from the same people who were questioning what I was going to do with my life!

I just blocked it out. I was adamant that this was it. Honestly, I had tunnel vision and didn't care what anyone thought. I hadn't been this fired up in a long time and it felt great.

Then, all of a sudden, all the coursework arrived. Loads of books and CD's for home learning before the practical in-person courses. My anxiety returned and it was crippling.

A negative dialogue began to run through my

mind: "Who am I to even think I could do something like this? I'm overweight. I used to be a nightclub promoter, how am I going to teach fitness?"

The anxiety had returned full whack and it was starting to affect my sleep again. I had suffered insomnia in the recent past which had really affected my life. It put strain on my partner, who although loving and devoted, was feeling the heat with my changing emotions.

I ended up getting sleeping pills from the doctor. With regards to my course, I was already booked in for practical weekends. I contacted the course provider to see if I could delay attending. As soon as I had a chat with them and explained honestly that I was suffering from anxiety, they told me it was totally fine to defer it for a few months. This instantly put my mind at ease.

My sleeping patterns thankfully returned. This made me realise that the root cause of my anxiety was due to the stress about becoming a personal trainer.

After a few weeks of sleeping better and my anxiety settling, I plucked up the courage to contact the course provider and book my first weekend course.

The anxiety and insomnia returned.

However, this time I was determined to battle on. I wanted a better life for myself. I didn't want to wake up at the age of thirty without a solid career. Besides, I had already committed financially to the course.

Driving from Cardiff to Bristol on a boiling hot Friday night in July 2006, I checked in at a Bed and Breakfast. It was the night before my first in-person module.

I barely slept a wink.

I tossed and turned all night. By 5am, the sunlight was streaming through the windows.

Fear gripped me. What if everyone else on the course was only eighteen years old, ripped and beautiful? They'd look at me; twenty-six and out of shape. They'd be thinking: "What the fuck is he doing here?"

I can't tell you how close I was to not attending that day. It would have been so easy to just drive straight home again, but something inside told me to face my fears.

I showered and continually splashed my face with cold water before heading out to Park Street for my course. It was 7.30am and I'd had about one hour's sleep.

Although early in the morning, it was already roasting hot. I was sweating and disheveled.

As I turned into the little street where the course was taking place, I noticed a guy in the distance. He was an absolute mountain of a man with a huge set of calves and a ruck sack over his shoulder. He was wearing the full sports get-up.

'Well, there's only one place he's going!' I thought. 'He must be going to the fitness course.' My immediate thoughts were: 'He's a hell of lot bigger than me!'

Despite my anxiety, I called over to him: "Hey mate, are you off to the fitness course?"

He turned around, plastered a big welcoming smile on his face and, in a deep West country accent, replied: "Yeah, I am! I'm heading to the course!" He held out his hand for me to shake it and introduced himself as Daryl.

Daryl, if you are reading this (we are still in touch), you will never know how much that meant to me.

Right there, in that moment, a ton of my anxiety disappeared. Moments later when I entered the room, all my fears were gone!

There must have been about twenty five or thirty people on the course. Yes of course, some of them were younger than me and in awesome shape, but there was such a mixed bag of people there. There were kids fresh out of college and there was a man in his sixties. We were all shapes and sizes.

I suddenly realised that all my fears prior to this moment were completely untrue.

Once everyone introduced themselves, I could see that they were normal people just like me; people who were hoping to change career and do something they felt passionate about.

I had a chat with the course provider during the break. Admitting my nerves, I told him about the worries I'd had about changing career at the age of twenty-seven. I firmly believed I would be the oldest and most out-of-shape in the room.

Amazingly, he told me that he was forty-years-old when he changed his career! From that moment on, my anxiety and insomnia disappeared.

Due to my lack of sleep that day, I somehow got through it on sheer adrenaline alone. By the end of the day, I was absolutely exhausted. Returning back to my B&B, I drank one beer and then slept soundly, straight through the night.

The following morning, I woke up refreshed

and relieved. Not only that, I felt enthusiastic to face the second day. I absolutely loved every moment of it.

Driving back to Cardiff on the Sunday night, I felt overwhelmed with joy, relief and happiness. Finally, I had focus for my future and most importantly, I was anxiety free.

I had almost allowed the fear to overcome me. Somehow, I had managed to face the fear, push through it and come out the other side. It was so liberating and it set me free.

I have since heard the term **FEAR** described as:–

False
Evidence
Appearing
Real

This could not ring more true. For months, I had built up a scenario in my head. I had imagined how the course would be and what the other people would be like. It was all totally false!

By overcoming this fear, I went on to complete my personal training diploma. There was a mixture of home-learning and in-person weekend modules. It took eight months and I loved every moment of it.

I shudder to think what would have happened if I didn't turn up that day; if I had got in my car and driven home again. The constant voices in my head told me I wasn't good enough. It almost made me turn back. Who knows what my life would have been like today?

Fitness not only changed my life, but it saved my life. I like to think I have then gone on to have a positive effect on others.

Perhaps you are reading this and feeling a bit lost in your career. Maybe you are thinking that you're too old and it's too late to change.

I'm telling you it's <u>NOT</u> too late.

I don't care if you're 30 plus, 40 plus, 50 plus or 60 plus; if you are unhappy where you are, you have the power to change it!

Nobody is going to give you permission. Nobody is going to do it for you.

In this day and age, with all the technology we have, opportunity is everywhere!

Ask yourself, what's the alternative?

Do you really want to settle where you are now?

If the answer is <u>NO,</u> then I hope this lights a fire within you to change.

Please don't allow yourself to look back in twenty years' time and say to yourself, 'I could have done that or I would have done that or I should have done that.'

Don't settle for mediocrity!

I'm not telling you to quit your job and walk out now. I'm telling you that you have an opportunity to explore other options.

It was February 2006 when I had my eureka moment. By December 2006, I was a fully qualified personal trainer.

I worked on my studies alongside my courier job. That meant I was still earning while studying. If I can do it, you can too!

By January 2007, I was equipped with flyers (a marketing tool that used to work in the nightclub days!) and a website (I think I paid £150 for it). I had even managed to get myself a ranking on Google under 'Cardiff personal trainers'.

I decided I would still work as a courier whilst building up a client base. Initially, I trained friends and family in the evenings and weekends.

I wasn't in a major rush to quit my courier job. I told myself that even if it took two years to build up my business, I was okay with that. The fact that I had focus and enjoyed what I was doing, was the most important thing.

With a spring in my step, a positive attitude and a flyer drop, I had built my business up within six months. I had some success with Google Ad words (no Facebook back then!) and I had gained eighteen hours per week with clients. I was finally able to quit the courier job and go full time.

In the space of just eighteen months, I had totally changed career. My life was heading in a brand-new direction, all because I made the decision to face my fears.

I tell you this, not to try to impress you. Rather, to try to impress upon you the importance of taking action.

My initial business was called 'Fitness and Motivation.' Back in the day, when I was a nightclub promoter, my house and garage brand was called 'Funkin' Marvellous'. I really wanted to stick with the 'FM' branding.

I became very busy, very quickly. Before I knew it, I was doing between 35-45 hours a week of personal training.

Now here's the interesting thing: Upon changing my career, I had never once considered how much money I could earn in fitness. I simply wanted to do something I was passionate about. Hand-on-heart, I'd never considered money.

Alongside this, my long-term partner and I split up, after almost a decade together. My previous anxieties had taken its toll. Despite the fact I was on a new trajectory, I'm not sure my partner thought it would last. We had also gotten older, developed different interests and simply started to drift apart.

As I approached thirty years old and single, I had the time to dive head-first into my business, often coaching seven days a week.

All of a sudden, I was earning a few quid. In fact, it was a lot more than before and I ended up buying an Audi TT sports car. It was a massive step-up from the courier days of being a white van man.

Despite being in the fitness industry for a few years, I'd held on to that white van. I'd arranged for a sign to be sprayed along the side: 'Fitness and Motivation'.

I did a lot of home visits at the time, so it was perfect for keeping my equipment in. There was a Swiss-ball, boxing gloves, bands and dumb-bells.

After the break up with my long-term partner, I moved in with a good mate Lee, who was a car salesman. He told me he could get me an Audi TT for a reasonably priced monthly figure. It said it would be a babe magnet!

He did and it was! ☺ zzzsmile

Despite loving my new life and being very happy in work, I was extremely busy. Too busy, in fact.

I would often down tools and spend the weekend at my Nan's house (God rest her soul) in the Forest of Dean. It was during this time that I started to think about how I could achieve a better work-life balance.

It was all great at the moment, but what if I had a family some day? Would I really want to be working late every night and seven days a week?

I'd been listening to some fitness gurus in the States who were talking about boot camps. They said you could train more people in one go; charge less and work less hours. I'd also been listening to a guru who said that you should become an expert in a certain 'niche' to really become the expert in your field.

All of this was bubbling around in my head. And then, back in early 2010, I had another 'Eureka!' moment – four years on since having the first one.

I was thirty-one years old, living with my friend Lee and feeling leaner and lighter than ever. It was a stark contrast to how I felt in my twenties, when I was battling my weight.

I was energized, clear-headed, no longer anxious, enjoying weight training and getting into kettle bells. I no longer felt I had to run myself into the ground for fat loss.

Then, 'Boom!' it hit me!

I wonder how many men of a similar age feel like I did?

Maybe, because they're on the wrong side of thirty, they feel their best days are behind them?

Personally, I feel great! It's a revelation how I feel at this age, especially because I felt overweight for years.

Taking action on my 'Eureka!' moment, I logged on to Facebook and put up a post: "I'm looking for ten Cardiff men over the age of thirty who feel their best days are behind them. I may have something for you." I also emailed all the mates I used to play five-a-side with.

Eight lads turned up at the old 'Train Station 2' gym in Cardiff. '30+Bootcamp' was born.

I am hoping that this book sparks a little fire within you. Perhaps you came here for fitness and fat loss. Maybe you will leave with not only that, but a career change?

Just one 'Eureka!' moment can change the trajectory of your life forever.

CHAPTER SIX

Accepting you are where you are

IN ORDER TO GET STARTED, you must first acknowledge where you are now.

Clients sometimes get angry or emotional after we have calculated their measurements. I calmly say to them: "You are where you are."

When you weigh and measure yourself, or take photos with your shirt off, it draws a line in the sand. Before, your head was simply buried in the sand, now you're facing facts.

Before we start with those measurements, let's talk about whatever it is that brought you to reading this book.

Back in 2019, I was on a dream holiday in Turkey with my family. Whilst lying by the pool, earphones in, I discovered some amazing audio by life coach Tony Robbins.

Tony Robbins is probably the world's most famous life coach. He deals with personal growth, business and relationships. However, this audio was about getting in shape. It was titled: 'The body you deserve'. It was actually aimed at women, but I was still very intrigued.

It really, really resonated with me. I've often told clients: "You don't need a new diet; you need a new mind-set." Everything Tony was talking about just confirmed this for me.

Even though I'd been into self-development for years, he gave me a different way of looking at things; things I'd like to share with you.

He asked the question "How long have your issues with food been controlling you?"

This was MASSIVE.

Then he said: "Are you prepared to let it control you for as long as it already has?"

Again, this was a HUGE question.

He went on, "Ask yourself: How many years have you been tolerating whatever is going on with your fitness, your health and your body?"

How many times have you started, sabotaged, then stopped?

How long have you been caught in this perpetual cycle, which you simply can't get out of?

Now ask yourself: how has this affected my life to date?

Have you turned down social occasions because you don't feel comfortable in your own skin? I know I have!

I've been that guy that said 'no' to going somewhere, simply because I thought I was going to be judged about my weight.

I've even gone as far as creating scenarios in my head. I'd imagine that people are already judging me based on my own poor perception of myself!

If you're nodding your head in agreement, I understand. Many, many clients have felt like this!

How else has it affected your life?

Have you refused to go out for meals with friends because you just don't feel comfortable in yourself? Maybe you've told yourself you won't be able to eat anything anyway because you are dieting?

Have you refused to take your kids swimming because you don't want to take your top off?

Have you refused to go to the beach and come up with something like: "I just don't like sand!" That was a favourite excuse of mine. In reality, I just panicked about having to take my top off. I felt, and looked, like a bag of shit.

Honestly, ask yourself how long this has been going on? You'll see it's been controlling your life and you may not have realized.

Looking at my own life, I realised that it had been controlling me from an early age. I started to get fat at the age of ten. I was using food as a comfort blanket for loneliness. We had moved house, away from all of the friends I used to play football with.

I then carried these bad habits and behaviors around with me, which in turn led me into the fitness industry. I wanted to learn how to fix myself. However, just getting into the fitness industry wasn't enough.

Yes, I fixed myself, but it was only temporary. In fact, the message from my earlier years in the industry has a LOT to answer for. In some ways, it only highlighted the issues I already had. I know this is the case for many others too.

It was only two years ago that I was listening to that Tony Robbins audio. I was forty years old and at the time, I'd say I felt okay. Not great, and better than I had been at points, but still just okay.

I thought: Wow! This has literally been my life! It has been controlling my behavior, on and off for thirty years!

Tony asked: "Are you prepared to let it control you, for the same time that it already has done, for the rest of your life?" That hit me really hard. It means I would be seventy years old and still fighting the same battle!

Why the hell would I want to be fighting this for the next thirty years?

That really punched me in the feels. It made me go inside and look at my own behavior in more depth.

You see, we all think we have time. We all think we can 'start again on Monday', but the truth is, time is running out.

Albert Einstein said: "Insanity is doing the same thing over and over again and expecting a different result."

Yet, I've done this multiple times. I'm sure you have too.

I don't want you to go to the grave still trying to figure this stuff out.

Think that sounds crazy? I've lost two clients who were good friends during this pandemic; not to COVID, but due to the fact that their lifestyle caught up with them. When they went to the grave, they had still been trying to find a way to lose weight and become healthier.

However, they simply weren't accepting the fact that it was their current behaviors that led to their ill health. They literally went to the grave still trying to crack it.

So, ask yourself this once more:

- Are you going to let this control you for the rest of your life?
- If so, then how is it going to affect your family life?
- Will you continually body-swerve trips to the beach?
- Will this behavior impact your kids? What about all the memories you could make?
- Are you going to continually say NO to taking your kids swimming because you don't want to take your top off?
- Are you going to keep making excuses NOT to go to the park with your kids because you feel like crap? These moments are surely what life should be about, right?
- Will you always lack spontaneity?
- What if a friend calls and invites you out somewhere? Do you instantly decline because you think you're going to feel uncomfortable due to your weight?

Listen, I know how you feel, I've been there.

I've turned down multiple occasions to go to things like school reunions because I didn't want people to think: "Oh Tregs, you've put on a bit of weight."

I've refused nights out because I couldn't find a shirt that fitted.

It's draining, it's exhausting and it controls you!

Now you can see it, it's time to break free from this prison. It's time to be released from the shackles of self-sabotage, forever.

I want you to forget about starting and stopping and putting a time cap on this.

Forget 28 days, 35 days, a few months…

We need to think beyond that. I want you to learn how to play this game for the rest of your life!

There is no wagon. There is no 'on' or 'off'. You simply just play the game for life. It's boring, it's not sexy, it's not going to wow you, but it will change your fucking life.

It's not aggressive, it's not radical; it's simply sustainable.

You will be amazed at just how simple this is.

CHAPTER SEVEN

Ask yourself: Why do I keep failing?

YOU MAY HAVE PURCHASED THIS BOOK looking for the 'magical' fat loss method. Perhaps you're hoping for a quick result.

Whilst I could easily give you some tips for a quick result, it would highly likely result in you going backwards once achieved.

If it's stopping and starting that's brought you here, then it's time to change that. It starts with no longer looking for the quick fix.

It's also going to take some deeper, (what I call 'inner work') to help change your identity, otherwise you will continue to fail in your attempts.

As I have already said: 'You don't need a new diet, you need to upgrade your mind-set'. That is why we need to cover this, before we even get into the health and fat loss.

I could give you access to the best trainers and

nutritionists in the world, but until you take a look at <u>WHY</u> you have continuously failed in the past, you will ultimately be stuck. We need to understand the 'why' before we move forward.

So why have you failed?

For me there are three major factors at play here.

As I break each once down, I will talk about my own experiences and how I came to understand and tackle them.

Factor 1 – Environmental conditioning

We are a product of our environment.

A sentence so profound yet something that is overlooked by so many.

A book I read recently called 'Atomic Habits' by James Clear stated that: 'Your environment is the hidden hand that shapes human behavior'. Another profound sentence that many of us would have failed to consider.

I realized how critical environment was, once I started to do inner work and went through counselling (Cognitive Behavioral Therapy). When my kids were young, I felt overwhelmed and shattered; unable to keep up with the message I was promoting in my business.

I grew up in a Gloucester with my mum. My parents were separated and I saw my dad most weekends. We lived in a maisonette in a place called Tuffley.

It was literally next door to my primary school, which was awesome. I could walk out the front door when I heard the bell and still not be late! Added to that, all my mates lived only a few minutes away. Some of my fondest memories are of kicking a football around every evening in the local field with my mates.

As a Manchester United fan, I was always pretending to be Bryan Robson or Mark Hughes. I stayed out until it got dark or mum called me in. I loved it.

However, around the age of nine or ten, mum bought a house with her new partner and we moved to a place called Robinswood, which was about four miles away.

'No big deal', you may think, but to a nine-year-old whose only mode of transport was a BMX bike, it was a massive change.

Don't get me wrong, I didn't hate it. In fact, the new house was bigger with a decent garden and in an okay area. It was just the fact that I could no longer meet my mates after school for a kick about.

I replaced with this with playing on my computer. I had an Atari 65xe with games like centipede and original football manager. As soon as I got home from school, I would play games and eat.

As an only child, there was no-one I had to share food with. There was also easy access to the cupboards. Mum worked late, so there was no-one to tell me to wait for my tea.

I started to gain weight.

Getting chubby as a ten-year-old isn't fun and I didn't like it. However, I had no idea that I using food for comfort. It was a coping mechanism to help me deal with not seeing my friends each evening.

Now I have to say, that none of this was particularly traumatic, in fact, nothing of the sort. I'm just explaining to you how my battle with food started with a change of environment.

I would never have known this until I tracked back during counselling to see where this pattern emerged.

It had taken me a few months to pluck up the courage to go and see a counsellor. I was 'Coach Tregs', owner and founder of '30 Plus Men's Fitness' with a rapidly growing successful boot camp and online business. I had moved to a beautiful house in the Vale of Glamorgan with my partner Sarah. On paper, things were great.

I was building a six-figure business, doing something I loved and developing a unique brand. However, things had moved very quickly for my partner Sarah and me. We now had two very young boys with only a sixteen-month age gap.

Sarah and I met in 2011 and after only a few dates, we had practically moved in with each other. It turns out we were living only two miles apart and she was actually training at the same gym I coached at!

After a few months, I gave up my flat and moved in with her. Shortly later, she fell pregnant with John. We were both elated. With both of us being over thirty, having children was something we had talked about early on in our relationship.

With a little one on the way and three cats, we quickly had to re-think living in an apartment overlooking the marina.

We were lucky to find a great place on a farm in the Vale of Glamorgan and moved in, barely a year after we had met. Our first-born was due just a few months later.

John came into this world on 13th August 2011, after a 37-hour labour. Sarah ended up having an emergency C-section. When John was handed to me, what should have been the best moment of my life quickly turned to horror.

The nurses whipped him away from me in a heartbeat. He was struggling for air having suffered from meconium aspiration (swallowing your own faeces). He was put on c-pap to aid breathing and then moved to an incubator.

He remained in ICU for three weeks and to say it was a troubling time, is an understatement.

No parent should ever have to experience the heartache of leaving the hospital without their baby, but that's exactly what we were told to do.

They were frightening times. We were told that John had some kind of lung issue. It was touch-and-go for a while. We even met the resident hospital chaplain to pray for him.

When we finally got to bring him home, he was far from one hundred per cent. He hadn't even been given the all-clear, but the doctors thought he might thrive at home with his parents.

On top of the nerves of being first time parents, we were given all sorts of equipment to monitor his breathing. It was extremely nerve-wrecking and stressful. It's fair to say that we really struggled. With the constant visits to and from hospital for check-ups, we never really got a solid routine going.

John was a terrible sleeper, but for the most part I wasn't too affected. My partner was breastfeeding and decided it would be best if she took the nights. However, most days she would end up messaging me, asking when I was coming home. She was at her wits end!

Sometimes, I would do the entire night shift with John and get zero sleep. Then I'd go to work, surviving on caffeine only. It was absolutely brutal!

I had gotten into pretty good shape before John was born. I knew my sleep and training would suffer when he arrived. Boy, was I right! Despite this, I managed to stay in okay shape.

After eight months of zero sleep and my missus losing her mind, I hired a specialist nanny to come in for a few days to help John get into a routine. She basically implemented what we were too tired to do. By the time she left, John was napping and sleeping loads better!

We were able to organize our first real date night in eight months. Finally, we could have some quality time together. I could hardly contain my excitement!

And then, all of a sudden, baby number two was on the way.

Let's just say, we were both freaked out, although naturally, my missus was much more terrified than me. She will be the first to admit that the second pregnancy was brutal, especially with a new-born at home.

Elliot came into the world on 17th January 2014 via a planned C-section. All of a sudden, it was double trouble.

Despite getting John into a better routine, with two young toddlers now at home, it was chaos. Double the shitty nappies, double the spew, double the screaming, double the stress.

We were both extremely overwhelmed, exhausted and completely balls-deep in parenthood. You have to remember, we had only met three years before and were still getting to know each other!

Added to this, with a growing business, I had bigger outgoings; much bigger in fact.

A couple of years before, I was living in a two-bed apartment in the Bay and driving an Audi TT. I was sleeping in and taking afternoon naps. I could come and go as I pleased. I was building a dream business with plenty of spare cash left over at the end of each month. Now, things were completely different.

Two kids under sixteen months old; a missus who was struggling and had given up her job; a bigger house; expensive council tax; staff to pay; running two cars (even though the TT went!) and about register for VAT! It's fair to say, the pressure was firmly on!

Around this time, I could really feel myself struggling with my training and eating habits.

I was determined to be able to train like I had done. I wanted to be as strict with my nutrition as I had been pre-kids, but it was quickly slipping away from me.

I vividly remember the talk I gave to myself one morning. After barely any sleep, I went downstairs, sank a load of coffee and told myself to 'man up and train'.

Going out to the front yard, I started on the kettlebell. After about fifteen swings, I dropped the bell, completely exhausted. I walked inside, went to the cupboard, found a packet of biscuits and devoured the lot. I felt like a complete fucking failure.

Around this time, I was always signed up to local races such as 10Ks and half marathons. Pre-kids, I was rocking up with a hangover and smashing a 10k in 42 minutes. A half marathon would take me only an hour and a half. Now, it was a completely different story. I didn't even have the energy to show up. On many occasions, I would drop out at the last minute and offer someone else my place.

It became a bit of a joke amongst my boot campers. The lads would say: "Don't worry about signing up. Tregs will give you his entry for free when he drops out the day before."

I tried to laugh it off and pretend to have the banter, but deep down, it hurt. The races that I had once loved and challenged myself with, were becoming something I no longer had the energy to even attempt.

However, things were about to get even tougher.

In December 2015, my eldest boy John slipped in the bathroom and broke his femur. I'd lifted him out of the bath and then went to reach for his brother. He tried to run off and slipped on the wet surface. A complete accident, but horrific all the same.

He spent weeks in hospital. Finally, he was allowed home, but he was strapped into a hip spica cast. It was down one full leg and half way down the other, which meant we had to wipe his bum through a flap in the cast! I'm chuckling as I write this, but looking back, it was hell!

We now had a baby (almost one years old) and a two-and-a-half-year-old toddler in a hip spica cast. Merry Fucking Xmas!

Thankfully, John made a full recovery and he's never had any issues since. However, just as he was getting back on his feet, we noticed that Elliot was in a lot of pain. He had been trying to walk and pull himself up on things, but recently, it seemed that he had retracted. He looked as though he was in constant pain with his neck bent to the side.

We thought it was an earache and gave him Calpol. However, his pain only continued to grow and we took him to hospital. He was put through a series of x-rays and invasive examinations to try to rule out anything sinister or neurological. He was diagnosed him with something called 'discitus' which was some kind of infection in the spine. Apparently, it had erupted after a recent bout of chicken pox. Elliot and Sarah ended up spending over a month in hospital!

Every day after coaching, I would collect John from nursery (another huge expense!) and we would head to hospital to see them. To save time, I'd often shove a burger into me at the hospital restaurant and sink back a pint to help cope with the stress.

Struggling to cope with the dramatic changes in my life, my sleep was poor, my stress was high and my eating was erratic. Added to that, some shit had gone down in my business, which compounded everything.

Two lads I had once called good friends, had set up a '30+ boot camp' franchise local to me. After a year, they decided they were going to re-brand and go it alone, taking a handful of my clients with them. Fucking nice one!

By the summer of 2015, business was booming, but I was really struggling personally. My online business was growing fast; so fast in fact, that I was even hosting seminars on how others could build an online business too.

However, at home it was just chaos. My missus and I were exhausted and the kids' routine was all over the place due to constant hospital visits. It seemed a never-ending conveyor belt of shitty nappies, spew and screaming. As much as I loved my kids, it was brutal.

In the week, I could hide out at the gym. I often sought the counsel of some of my older clients. They had been through everything I was going through.

However, it was the weekends where I felt I couldn't escape or switch off from the stress. Despite having to do a Boot camp on a Saturday morning, there were no other work commitments. I would teach boot camp; tired and groggy, but full of caffeine. Then, I'd dash into the bakery on the way home, picking up cakes and baguettes.

I'd end up eating crap and drinking beers during the weekend, but telling myself I'd go ultra 'clean' on Monday.

I'd wake up on a Sunday, puffy-faced and bloated with bags under my eyes. Exhausted and snappy, I'd end up diving head-first into sugary cereal. I was putting on weight and it was starting to become noticeable.

I started to think I might need help. Searching on the internet for local counsellors, I found one that dealt with addictions; drugs, alcohol, gambling, sex and of course, food. This looked like just what I needed. However, I procrastinated for about two months before I finally took the plunge and made contact.

My missus could see I was binging, but what was even more alarming, was the fact that my eldest son was starting to copy me. He would try to eat several packets of crisps back-to-back (a terrible habit I had developed). John was barely three years old, but he was creeping into the cupboards and sneaking multiple packets of crisps. It was when I realised my son was picking up my awful behaviors, that I knew it was time to take action.

I didn't really know what to expect from my first session, but it was such a relief being able to offload. I told my counsellor, Steven, that I was feeling like a fraud. I was building a business I loved, but simply could not stick to the 'clean-eating' message I was promoting.

About six weeks into our sessions, I had a massive break through. Steven had already been asking me questions about my life, but this time he tracked backwards through my past to highlight any events that stood out.

"Why do I have to do that?" I asked him.

He told me that quite often an incident may

have happened to send us off in a slightly different direction; perhaps the loss of a loved one, or some other trauma could trigger us in a negative way.

We started to look back to see where this bad relationship with food had begun. Why did I feel it was normal to eat five or six bags of crisps back-to-back? We tracked it all the way back and BANG, it hit me! It had begun, just like I said, when we had moved away from my friends.

That was when the weight gain had begun, because prior to that moment, food had never been an issue to me. In the subsequent months, Steven and I unraveled more bad habits. He told me that behaviors that have been developed or learned could be unlearned.

It was only when we started to unravel these issues, that I remembered what friends used to say to me. We'd be in the pub and they would comment: "Fucking hell Tregs, are you hungry? You've had a packet of crisps with every single pint!"

Honestly, I thought this was the norm. I brushed it off without giving it much thought. It was bad behavior that I had picked up through being at home alone and it had just developed over time.

Steven asked me: "Do you eat in secret?"

"What do you mean?" I asked, stalling for time.

"Well, if you have food and you don't want anyone to see you eating it, do you go into another room and eat it away from people?"

Boom! It hit me again! I'd been doing this for most of my adult life. I'd go to the shop to buy healthy food, but I'd end up picking up snacks and making sure I ate them in private before going home.

If you are nodding along because you've done the same, then I hope this gives you some insight.

With some more tracking back through my life, I recalled a time when mum came home with our usual Friday night fish and chips. I leapt up to hide a big plate of cheese and crackers behind the sofa. I didn't want her to catch me eating, because she'd know full well I'd been sneaking extra grub.

The insights from the counselling were incredible and over a period of eight months, I slowly started to change my relationship with food.

It was around that time that 'flexible dieting' was becoming popular in the industry. One day, Steve announced: "Tregs you don't need to come here anymore."

"Maybe not," I replied, grateful. "But this has given me so much self-esteem. I'll also be able to pass your insights on to my clients, so thank you."

I was being one-hundred honest; I had found it fascinating. The extra knowledge around human psychology allowed me to coach clients on a deeper level.

As I write this, I still have daily struggles with trying not to over-eat, but the crazy binges are a thing of the past. It feels so good to say this because at one time, I was really feeling like a lost cause.

If you are reading this and feeling like a lost cause, then I'm here to tell you that you are not! You can fix yourself with a little help. It takes time, but it is so worth it.

With all that said, I want you to stop for a minute and think about any poor behaviour you have with food. Track back through your life and ask yourself: Where did these begin? Can you identify anything?

After many conversations with Steven, and indeed with my clients, I can tell you that many of these behaviors are picked up as a child, simply due to environment.

One client said that her meal times as a kid were never fixed and often very erratic. She 'tracked back' and said that it sent a shiver down her spine. She re-visited the worry she had as a kid; not having a set meal time and wondering if they would get food that evening at all.

A close friend who has food issues said it began for her at boarding school. Why? Because there was a lock on the fridge. You couldn't access food, apart from at meal times. Therefore, if you didn't like what you were given, it was tough, you had to eat it. When you look at it, can you see how dangerous this can be?

I already told you my three-year-old son was starting to copy my behaviour by eating multiple packets of crisps back-to-back. He was simply following his dad's behavior!

Remember that sentence by James Clear at the start of this section? "Your environment is the hidden hand that shapes human behavior?"

Let's look at that.

Let's say you have told yourself that you'll start again on Monday. This is your week! Your meals are prepped and you're all set for the gym. The only thing is, your partner loves a mid-week takeaway. In fact, she also enjoys a few mid-week glasses of wine.

Halfway through the week, she starts calling you 'boring' because you don't want the takeaway. She says you're uptight because you're not having a beer.

It's only an example of course, but one I've heard hundreds of times over the years.

"You don't need to lose weight – I love you just the way you are," is another one that gets banded around when one partner is working on their fitness and the other isn't.

This is a massive factor that needs to be considered. Your environment must be conducive to your goals!

I've lost count of the number of times a client has said: "My partner is so unsupportive of my weight loss." It's something that needs to be addressed from the get-go.

Look, I'll be brutally honest with you here; I separated from a partner I had in my twenties because of this very issue. We met during my clubbing days when I was working as a music events promoter. The first three years of our relationship were all about partying. Then we moved in and got a little more sensible. Less weekend partying, but, combined with the mid-week drinks, partying was still a big part of our lives.

When I decided to become a personal trainer at the age of twenty-seven, I was really trying hard to be healthier. I wanted to stay at home more and focus on myself, rather than go out drinking. It did become a problem at times.

She would say things like: "All you want to do is eat boring meals and not drink. I want to have a glass of wine mid-week and let my hair down at the weekends."

It started to take its toll and although it's fair to say there were other factors affecting our relationship, the fact that we had changed socially did play a big part.

Now, if you're reading this and thinking: *'I'm going to have to leave my missus in order to lose weight!'* just chill for a second. Don't do anything hasty!

The fact that I've made you aware of how your home environment may affect you is crucial. We can address this now.

Firstly, I want you to understand that your partner does NOT have to be on the same journey as you and therefore you do NOT have to pressure them to do the same.

What you DO need to do however, is make them aware of how important it is for you to change.

Something as simple as saying: "Hey (name), I really want to make some positive changes to my health and fitness. I know you love me as I am, but I want to lose weight for me. I really believe this will have a positive effect on everyone. I'm not asking you to join me; I just hope you can support me on my journey."

That is just one example. Trust me, if your partner loves you, they will appreciate your efforts and want to support you. You'll need to sort out the logistics of food-shopping, cooking, meal-prep and meal times, but before you do, you'll need to have this conversation.

Now, if you have a partner who knows about your desire to change, but continues to make it an issue, then understand that the problem isn't with you; it's with them.

You see, loved ones can often feel threatened when a partner tries to better themselves and lose weight. It's simply because of their own securities; their fear of being 'left behind'.

Trust me when I say that the only reason

someone would try to bring you down, is because they feel threatened or insecure themselves.

It's a tricky one and I certainly don't have all the answers. I'm simply making you aware of something you may have to consider.

Whilst you don't have to powerfully impose your new lifestyle on your loved one, you can let your actions rub off on them, in a positive way. To give you an example, I want to tell you a little story.

Around twelve years ago, I had just come out of the long-term relationship I was talking about earlier. I moved in with Lee, a good friend of mine. We had met back in university, but remained great friends.

Lee was a car salesman. He was recently single too, earning a few quid and loving life. We were both in our early thirties and had been heavily into music and clubbing in our early twenties. By the time we moved in together, I had been working in the fitness industry for four years and living a healthy way of life. Lee was the opposite.

The first day we moved in together, Lee announced: "Tregs I'm going to take you down to the village tonight for a few pints and a burger."

Off we went, and it was great fun.

The next day, I was at the gym and Lee texted: "Indian tonight?"

I thought, *'Yeah fuck it, what the hell!'*

So that night, we had a massive Indian takeaway. No word of a lie, the next day he messaged me: "Chinese later?"

By then, I was thinking, *'Jeez, that's three nights of eating out on the trot!'* I wasn't used to it, but to be polite, I duly agreed.

By the end of the week, I felt about a stone heavier. The problem was real, and if this carried on, fun as it may be, I was going to balloon. It didn't help that Lee, despite having a poor diet, was very slim. His eyes were bigger than his fucking belly! He could barely finish a third of his takeaway before feeling full and pushing it away. Meanwhile, Mister 'issues with food' over here, would be waiting like a praying mantis, ready to polish off his leftovers!

I had to sit down with Lee and have a chat. I said: "Look mate, this is great fun, but as you know, I'm a personal trainer and I've had issues with my weight in the past. I really don't want to risk getting fat again."

Surprisingly, Lee replied: "Tregs, I know fuck-all about nutrition, but if you lead me by the hand, I'm happy to try a new diet. I could do with feeling a bit better, so I'll put my trust in you."

It was music to my ears! Subsequently, I went off and stocked up on loads of protein, veggies and fruit. I started to cook every evening, and although it was basic stuff like chicken or fish with stir-fry, Lee actually really enjoyed it. The good thing was, I hadn't imposed it on him. I had merely talked about my own diet and he wanted to give it a go! By simply having that one conversation early on, it made life a whole lot easier.

Here's the best bit. When I moved in with Lee, he had a conversation with me too.

"Tregs, I know you're lively and full of banter first thing in the morning, but I'm not a morning person. Please don't expect any chat out of me in the morning, it takes me a while to get going."

I chuckled to myself, but respected his wishes and stayed out of his way. It was true, he was a right misery-guts in the mornings!

However, weirdly, after about a week of cooking for him and giving him proper nutrition, there was a change. No word of a lie, I woke up one morning to hear this prick singing in the shower! He was even whistling as he put on his suit!

The more I cooked for him and made sure he drank his two litres of water a day, the more lively and happier he became.

"Tregs, I can't believe it! I've got so much more energy! I just thought I hated my job and lived for the weekends!"

"No, you daft prick!" I replied. "You've been undernourished and chronically dehydrated for years. No wonder you've been a misery!"

It just goes to show how environment can either control us or how we can learn to control it!

Willpower and motivation will only take you so far. If your house is filled with booze and unhealthy food, then you need to address that. Your home needs to be set up correctly, in order for you to win. I'm extremely lucky now that my indoors environment is set up for me to succeed.

My dad lives with us. He has two beers with his Sunday lunch and maybe one beer during the week if there's a match on. That's about it. My missus doesn't drink and she lives a healthy lifestyle. We've never really been 'takeaway' people. In the ten years we've been together, I think we've maybe ordered three takeaways in total. We're not dessert people. With two boys in the house aged seven and eight, we do have things like chocolate in the cupboards, but it's out of reach and doesn't come out often.

None of this is to impress you – I'm simply stating the facts.

We're the type who goes to bed early and it's lights out at 10pm.

Bloody hell, that sounds really boring, doesn't it? However, at forty-two years old, it suits me down to the ground. More importantly, it keeps me congruent with my goals of staying fit, lean and energized.

So, what about you?

Does you environment control you? Or are you in control?

Just sit and think about that for a second.

Is it time you sat down and had that conversation with a loved one?

Do you need to remove alcohol from the house?

Does this give you some food for thought before moving forward?

I really hope it does.

Factor 2 – You are "all-or-nothing"

We live in an age of the internet and Amazon prime. We can order something at the click of a button and it arrives within twenty-four hours.

We are surrounded by the diet culture: magazines and advertisements promise six-pack abs in twenty-eight days. As consumers, we buy into it! We want results and we want them now. Unfortunately, this mentality is only destined to make us fail.

Let's look at the post-festive season; January in particular. Half of the nation will embark upon new year's resolutions.

Whilst I'm no stranger to making a joke about the 'New Year, New me' crowd, I salute anyone who wants to improve their health and fitness.

The problem, especially in the new year, is that people impose massive expectations on themselves; not only from a training point of view, but with huge restrictions on nutrition.

Quite often, these 'targets' are set after the excesses of the festive period when people, quite frankly, feel like shit.

They tell themselves they are going to do x, y and z in order to quickly rid themselves of the excess weight. Herein lies a massive problem. A person may tell themselves they are going to hit the gym five times a week and restrict to a low-calorie intake.

It's easy to make these resolutions when you're sitting in a chair, beer in hand, eating cheese and watching Christmas movies. When it comes to putting the resolutions into practice, it's not that easy.

How do I know all of this?

I've been that guy!

Remember, my battle with weight started at the tender age of nine or ten and it was an ongoing battle. It's the thing which eventually lead me into the fitness industry to do a personal training diploma at the age of twenty-seven.

When I was only about twelve or thirteen, I had over-eaten at Christmas and felt like crap. I was probably in my first year of secondary school and had been introduced to the local cross-country route. We ran it during school hours, but I had also gone a few times on my own. I lived nearby and came up with a plan. On New Year's Day, I decided that I was going to run this (three or four mile) course not once, not twice, but three times in one day!

Yep, three runs in one day (accumulating to ten or twelve miles off-road) for a thirteen-year-old! One in the morning, one at lunch and one in the evening. In true 'New Year, New me' style, I decided to start on New Year's Day.

I didn't go back to school until say, the 5th or 6th January and I remember thinking that it would give me at least a week of training.

On New Year's Day I got up, laced up and went off on my four-mile run. It was difficult because I had gained some weight during Christmas, but I got through it.

I had a shower, something to eat and told myself I'd be off again in a few hours. That's exactly what I did. By early afternoon I was off again on my second cross-country run of the day. I'd never done two in a day before but there I was, aiming for three runs a day, for the next week!

I got the second run done and had my second shower and change of the day.

Then, when darkness fell on New Year's Day, I went out on my third cross-country run.

By the end of the day, a thirteen-year-old kid who had gained weight at Christmas, had ran three cross-country routes in one day. And the plan was to do it all over again the next day, or so I thought.

I woke up absolutely shattered and barely able to move. I was suffering with, what I now know is, severe DOMS (Delayed onset of muscle soreness).

I was in agony, but in my mind, I was still committed to three runs a day.

So, on the morning of 2nd January, I laced up and headed out for my fourth run in under twenty-four hours. It hurt, it sucked and I felt miserable.

If my memory serves me, I may have completed a second run that day, however I most certainly couldn't complete the third. By the end of the day, I was completely shattered and starving.

On day three (3rd January) I couldn't move. My 'healthy-eating' plan had gone out the window and I was so famished that I was hoovering up food like there was no tomorrow.

At the tender age of thirteen, I had made myself suffer by setting the most unrealistic and punishing goal. It was only going to end in failure and frustration.

Now you may be astounded to read this, perhaps even having a chuckle at my crazy behaviour. However, let me tell you, thousands of people set themselves up for failure every week, by imposing crazy demands on themselves.

Sure, they may not be stupid enough to tell

themselves they are going to run three times a day. However, telling yourself you are going to hit the gym four or five days a week when the last time you entered a gym was a year ago is just as destructive.

The same goes for doing super low-calorie diets; you are simply not going to be able to sustain this.

Even though I could tell you a hundred stories of clients going too hard and then subsequently crashing and burning, I'm going to pick the one that stands out the most for me. I think a lot of you are going to be able to resonate with this.

I've changed the guy's name out of respect. A few years ago, I met and trained a lad called Rob.

He was due to get married abroad in a year's time and wanted to look his best (a wedding is a massive motivation after all). Admittedly, he had a lot of weight to lose, but with a twelve-month time scale, he had given himself plenty of time.

As with all clients, I began to educate him about calories-in and calories-out (as I am will do with you later in this book). I also introduced him to intermittent fasting, which is a way of dieting where you simply skip a meal to help facilitate a calorie deficit. This is something I'll talk about later too.

Rob really absorbed this info and started to put it into practice. The problem was, he started to go too aggressive with it. He was doing 'fasted' cardio in the morning, extended 24-hour fasts and very low-calorie intakes.

He would come to the gym to train and he'd be enthusing about it all, but I could see it was going to be unsustainable in the long run.

I advised him: "Rob, you're going too aggressive. You won't be able to sustain it. You're gonna crash and burn mate. It won't end well."

He said he was just fine; that with the amount of weight he wanted to lose, he had to really go for it.

He kept mentioning the wedding and how it was keeping him focused. Well, to cut a long story short, Rob lost six stone in one year!

He was doing a lot of work on his own, but on the one or two times I saw him during the week, I tried to continually advise him. "Rob you can eat more food and your diet can be more varied bud. It doesn't have to be bland meals."

He insisted that he had it all under control.

Rob got married and the weight loss was there for all to see. He looked like a different bloke. After his wedding, we lost touch for a bit. Then some months later, he messaged me and we got chatting. When I asked him how he was, he admitted that he'd put some weight back on. He said that he would get it sorted soon.

Six months passed before he messaged me again. He had put all the weight back on.

His words were something like: "Mate, I just can't stop eating! I feel like shit! Every morning when I wake up, I tell myself I'll sort it, but the next thing I'm ordering another takeaway. I just can't stop."

What had happened to Rob was something that many fail to consider when they go all-or-nothing. There was a massive psychological rebound.

This is why I tell you that you don't need a new diet; you just need to fix your mind-set.

Despite my consistent warnings, Rob had gone too hard.

Fair play to him, because he kept up the super-strict regime for longer than most. The wedding was, after all, a major focus for him, but after the big day, it all came crashing down.

Is any of this resonating with you? I'm sure it is.

I remember a chat I had with another client.

She told me how she had read a book about binge eating and she recited a paragraph to me: "Imagine you swim under-water for ninety seconds. When you come up for air, you're not going to take a little breath. You're going to take a massive gulp of air because you haven't had any for ninety seconds."

What happens if you go on a super-strict diet for a sustained period of time, cutting out all your favorite foods? When you finally achieve your goal, will you cave in, eating all the treats you have been denying yourself?

Are you just going to have just the one biscuit or are you going to eat the entire packet? I think we all know the answer.

In my fifteen years of coaching, I've had thousands of conversations with clients about extreme diets they have tried.

There's 'Herbalife' (shake for breakfast, shake for lunch, evening meal), 'Keto' (high fat, moderate protein, zero carbs), 30 days no sugar (exactly what it says on the tin) – the list goes on.

People say, "Well, it worked for me, I lost loads of weight!"

I then ask them, "Yes, but what happened after?"

To which, they sheepishly reply, "I put it all back on!"

So, it begs the question, did it really work? Or did it just mess you up psychologically in the long term?

Sometimes a person will try to revisit the 'extreme' diet they had great results with in the past, only to find that the second time around, they simply cannot stick to it.

The first time around, their motivation was high, but the second time around, they remember just how much it sucks. They end up throwing the towel in much quicker.

What follows is the feeling of failure, possibly a binge, and the dreaded cycle continues.

Please understand this, if you go too hard, you are doomed for failure. You have no idea of the psychological damage you are doing to yourself.

Life is stressful enough with kids, jobs and careers, not to mention a bloody pandemic! Why on earth would you want to add more stress into the mix by going on an extreme diet?

Factor 3 – You have poor self-image and believe you don't deserve it

The third factor is again a psychological one and

extremely difficult to crack. However, if you truly want to break free from whatever is holding you back, then you need to work on this. It's easier said than done of course, but it is possible with time, effort and practice.

Later in this book, I will talk about the Law of Attraction and how it changed my life. However, for now, without getting too spiritual, I want to cover one of the greatest things it taught me: 'self-talk'.

As humans, we are always thinking. We can be thinking good things, bad things, positive or negative, but we are always thinking.

Our thoughts can be influenced by many external factors such as our environment, people around us, the media and so on. It's important to really understand that our thoughts control us. However, quite often, our thoughts are influenced by what we see and here.

As well as having thoughts, we also talk to ourselves. What do I mean by this?

Well, have you ever looked at yourself in the mirror and called yourself a 'fat bastard'? I know I have.

Have you ever gone shopping and tried on clothes, only to feel completely uncomfortable in them? Did you tell yourself something like: 'Who am I kidding trying to wear this? I look like shite! I'll never be able to pull this off!'

I have.

Have you ever thought about entering a physical challenge and then the internal dialogue pipes up: 'You can't do that! What makes you think you can do that? You're not good enough or fit enough!'

I have.

If you're reading this and nodding in agreement, then you're not alone.

Just stop for a second and ask yourself: would you let a friend talk to you like that?

Would you let a loved one call you 'fat' and 'worthless'?

I think we know the answer, right?

So why would you talk to yourself like it?

You can change the negative self-talk, but first you need to understand where it comes from.

Your conscious mind controls the practical stuff like brushing your teeth, driving your car and walking to your office – things which you do on autopilot without giving it much thought.

Then there's your subconscious mind. Your subconscious mind has no ability to reject signals and it has been absorbing messages ever since you were a child.

Perhaps your parents told you that you weren't good enough, time and time again? Perhaps it stuck? Maybe an ex-partner called you 'fat' and it stuck.

Perhaps friends have joked about your weight and it stuck.

These words have become absorbed into your subconscious mind and you have accepted them. You have even started to talk to yourself like that and now it's the message on replay throughout your mind.

You may not have even considered this until now, but every time you started on a health and fat-loss kick, subconsciously you believed you were going to fail.

You might get so far, even lose a little weight, perhaps even achieve your goal for a short while, but then it all comes crashing down. You go back to where you started, thinking that you'll never crack it. You end up feeling like there's simply no point.

Before I give you training and diet protocols, we need to create your new self-image, otherwise you'll be perpetually destined to fail.

We are going to revisit how to change this negative self-talk and image later on in the book when we cover the Law of Attraction.

We'll get into the practicalities and the nitty-gritty of how to get healthy, lose fat and keep it off. I will equip you with the essential tools of how to do this the right way. We'll then go back to changing the internal dialogue.

For now, I just want to touch on this subject and make you realise that you're not alone.

CHAPTER EIGHT

The Ultimate Factors –
Hydration and Sleep

BEFORE I GIVE YOU THE 'GOLD' and teach you about calories, protein, exercise and how to put it all together, I am going to break down what I call the two ULTIMATE factors.

I have often said that if I had just one minute to give someone my best bits of advice for health and fat loss, then it would be hydration and sleep.

I literally cannot stress enough that without these two factors taken care of, everything else will be so much harder to implement.

Plain and simple, if you aren't sufficiently hydrated, then you won't feel (or perform) anywhere near as good as you could.

Likewise, if you have continuously poor sleep, then you won't feel (or perform) anywhere as near as good as you could.

Added to that, hunger, mood, willpower and

decision-making will also be negatively affected.

When I say that hydration and sleep really are the ULTIMATE factors, then they really are the ULTIMATE FACTORS.

Let's start with the easiest one to master.

HYDRATION

It wasn't until the age of about twenty-two, that I finally understood the importance of being hydrated. I had gone on (what was to be a dream) holiday to the Cayman Islands, with my girl-friend at the time.

My mum, who had previously worked on cruise ships, had been living there for a year. She invited us to go and stay with her for three weeks. It was going to be a dream holiday and we couldn't wait.

At that age, I was in a perpetual cycle of yo-yo dieting. My behaviour with food was erratic, but I wasn't fully aware of it at the time. I had joined the gym at the nearby Marriot hotel and was going three times a week with my mates.

Bear in mind, I was completely clueless at the time. My routine would generally be three sets of everything (upper body only), and then go and have a sauna!

Whilst I got quite into it, I had no clue about nutrition. I was eating everything in sight, assuming I would bulk up.

Prior to this, I had only really been into running, but I grew frustrated with it due to injuries. Now that I had stopped running and started (half-arsed) upper body lifting, I was eating more and gaining weight rapidly.

Looking back, I couldn't see it. I lacked so much self-awareness back then.

It wasn't until a few days before I was going on holiday that it hit me.

I went into town to buy some T-shirts for my break. Whilst I normally wore a large, I was shocked to discover that large was too tight and I needed extra-large!

I'd been telling myself I was getting muscular, but the truth was I had put on a LOT of body fat.

It was too late now though. I went on the long-haul flight and for the first time ever, I was really sweating and getting quite smelly.

I'm sure this has happened to a few of you guys on flights or public transport? It's not a nice feeling, right?

Well after one long-haul flight and one internal flight, we touched down in the beautiful

Cayman Islands. As soon as the cabin doors of the aircraft swung open, boom! The heat and humidity hit me.

Fuck, it was hot and I felt really uncomfortable.

I had told my mum over the phone that I had been hitting the weights and gotten bigger, however she hadn't seen me in person for a while. I could see the look of shock across her face when she saw me.

"Wow!" she said. "You have really beefed up!"

I knew she was just trying to be polite.

The first day that we headed outside, I put on a vest. I thought I'd look awesome because of all the curls I'd been doing, but actually, I just felt like a fat blob.

The next day we went to the beach and when I took my top off, I felt truly disgusted in myself. I honestly couldn't believe how shit I looked.

Looking back at the pictures of the holiday only confirmed it.

The heat was unbearable. I had never experienced heat like it and, at my heaviest weight ever, it was seriously uncomfortable. I was sweating badly and having some really bad body odor. It was awful.

Meanwhile, my girlfriend at the time happened to be in great shape and was a bit of a looker. I can't tell you how inferior I felt next to her.

She drew a fair bit of attention around the pool and pretty much everywhere we went. In my head, I was constantly telling myself that all these other blokes must be looking at her and thinking: *'What is she doing with a fat bastard like him?'*

There I was, on a stunning island, staying free of charge at my mum's. I was with my beautiful girlfriend for three weeks in glorious tropical sunshine and yet I felt miserable.

Of course, I didn't let on. I enjoyed experiences such as snorkeling in amazing clear blue sea, brunching at posh hotels and hanging out in cool bars with my mum's friends. However, it was all tarnished by my inward misery about how I looked and felt.

I told myself I'd never allow myself to feel so shit on holiday again, but of course I did. If you've ever felt fat on a beach holiday in blazing hot temperatures, then you'll know all too well what I'm talking about.

I asked my mum if there was a gym I could use nearby. I still really wanted to train. Thankfully, there was an awesome 'Gold's gym' and I got a three-week pass.

I could see I was in shit shape. I had been focusing purely on upper body. Also, because I was overweight with skinny calves, I would get calf strain if I attempted a run! Talk about being in a right state, eh?

To make matters worse, this gym was fucking serious. Even though Cayman was a small island, the gym was filled with proper lifters. They were all tanned and bronzed and the women were in seriously sexy shape.

On the one hand, it compounded my misery, but on the other hand, it was very inspiring.

After about a week of going to Gold's Gym, I noticed an advert for a one-to-one consultation with a nutritionist.

Realising that whatever I had been doing hadn't worked, I decided to book a consultation for an hour.

For the first ten minutes, I poured my heart out to the lovely American lady. I told her about all the training I did and how I was much more active than any of my mates. I complained that I didn't understand how I could still feel so fat. Before I could protest any longer, she interrupted me.

Placing a two-litre bottle of water on the table, she said: "Okay, so how much of this are you drinking a day?"

I thought: *'Jeez, I've just poured my heart out to you and all you can do is ask me how much water I'm drinking?'*

However, I stopped for a moment to consider her question. Then I replied: "Well, we have a water cooler fountain in the office at work (I was a music event promoter at the time). I probably have two cups a day. The rest is diet coke."

She nodded her head, as though it was all coming together in her mind. She then went on to ask me what colour my pee was! She wanted to know what colour it was 'most' of the time, and not just after I'd woken up.

Trying not to laugh at her question, I replied: "Yellow".

Nodding again, she told me I was severely dehydrated and that was why I felt so hungry. She said that most people confuse dehydration with hunger. She went on to tell me that if I drank a minimum of two litres of water a day, I would feel a massive improvement – not only in alertness, energy and skin complexion, but my digestion would improve and I would generally feel healthier.

"Water is the key to vitality," she said.

The advice she was giving m (although I couldn't grasp it at the time) was completely life changing. Learning about hydration changed my life, and quickly too.

We discussed many other things during the consultation which quite frankly, after twenty years I have forgotten, but the message about hydration remained.

I went away and immediately began upping my water. I started fresh bottled mineral water as the tap water wasn't recommended in the Cayman Islands.

My mum remarked that she had been alarmed to see me drink Diet Coke first thing in the morning. She was pleased to see me swapping to bottled water.

On a side note, Diet Coke has zero calories, so from a fat-loss perspective, you have nothing to worry about. I still enjoy the occasional Diet Coke today, but the bulk of my fluid intake is water.

Well, blow me down! I couldn't believe how

much different I felt in such a short period of time! Like, literally, forty-eight hours!

The best thing about getting hydrated is that it's fucking easy to do! You just drink water!

Now don't get me wrong, I was still fat and not liking my reflection in the mirror. I was also still on holiday so I was eating loads and boozing. However, when I woke up in the mornings, I would immediately start on the water.

My energy began to increase. That fuzzy feeling the morning after a few beers disappeared so much quicker. I <u>did</u> feel less hungry. Generally, I felt more positive with a better sense of get-up-and-go.

The nutritionist had told me that clear pee is a sign of hydration, so I became obsessed with getting my pee clear by midday!

When we left the Cayman Islands, despite not feeling good in myself on that holiday, I felt like I had been given an extremely powerful tool. Returning home, I embarked on a serious weight loss quest.

One year later, I went on another dream holiday with the same partner, this time to the Dominican Republic. I was three stone lighter and felt amazing.

Becoming hydrated had been a KEY component for this.

Now I have to be honest with you, this was NOT the end of my weight problems. My weight continued to go up and down over the years due to multiple different factors.

However, understanding the importance of hydration and knowing how drinking plenty of water can make you feel better in a short space of time, had a truly profound effect on my life.

From that point onwards, it didn't matter if I was on holiday with my feet up, drinking and eating what I liked or doing zero exercise, I would always do one thing: get hydrated.

Even if all other bets were off, I would always drink water from the moment I woke up in order to get my pee clear.

If you are reading this and have never focused on hydration, then I cannot stress the importance of this. In the past I would recommend one litre per 25kg of bodyweight, but if you are a heavier guy, I don't want you worrying about drinking five litres!

For me, two to three litres of clean water a day is more than sufficient to get you feeling energized, clear-headed and to keep unnecessary hunger at bay.

You might be thinking *'Is that it? Drink water?'*

All I will say is: give it a go and let's see how you feel within just a few short days.

Of course, that's NOT 'it', but it is one of my ultimate factors. If you get hydration right first, then you'll be able to follow the rest of the information I'm going to share with you.

SLEEP

Ultimate factor number two is something most men struggle with. There are many reasons for this, the main ones being: young children, erratic work schedules and work shifts. I've experienced them all!

I always tell clients I can't fix your sleep for you! Improving sleep is much harder than improving hydration, but I need you to understand just how bloody important good sleep is.

It's something that needs to be addressed before you start any training or nutritional programme. I guarantee it is so often overlooked with men of our age, so let's get into it.

I have always enjoyed my sleep and lots of it! For large parts of my life, I have slept very well. The only times I really struggled was during bouts of anxiety in my late twenties and during the first few years of my kids' lives.

Whilst I always enjoyed a sleep (and an afternoon nap) I never really began to understand the benefits of it, until I got into the fitness industry. What I began to learn was extremely enlightening and only made me want to sleep more!

The first major factor about sleep is that it can actually help you curb your appetite! Yes, that's right, good sleep can actually minimise your hunger.

You see, when we have a good night's sleep (and most men should aim for between 7-9 hours), we keep the hunger hormone 'ghrelin' at bay.

Ghrelin can be a real kicker if you are trying to lose weight. With it being a hunger hormone, it only makes you want to eat more food! Ghrelin is produced whenever we have a bad night's sleep!

Just stop for a moment and think about the days you have an early alarm. What about the days when you've had a bad night's sleep due to the kids waking you? Haven't you felt hungrier during the day? That, my friend, is ghrelin and it's very real!

Some guys can handle poor sleep and the

hunger that comes with it, but 90% of us can't – including yours truly. I gained two stone when my kids were young!

Of course, poor sleep doesn't pull calories out of thin air and pop them in your mouth! However, it does make you less disciplined and less motivated to stick to your diet, hence you are much more likely to over-eat.

Added to this, poor sleep can make you stressed. When you are stressed, you produce a hormone called cortisol. You'll be more likely to make bad nutrition decisions and over-eat.

When my kids were young, my partner and I suffered badly with lack of sleep. The sleep deprivation went on for about three years and it was hell. I was literally drowning in ghrelin and cortisol!

Added to this, I was trying to train as hard as I could before the kids came along. I was surviving off copious amounts of coffee and pre-workout drinks. I was beaten up, overweight and exhausted!

Stop for a moment and imagine you have been going around dehydrated and suffering from lack of sleep for years. Can you see why you have been failing time and time again?

- Dehydrated = lethargy and hunger
- Poor sleep = lethargy, hunger, poor willpower, poor motivation.
- = Combine these two together and you are in big trouble!

Can you see why I am addressing this before we even discuss exercise? After all, exercise is a big stressor on the body and if you are not hydrating or getting adequate recovery, then it is no use!

Talking of recovery, sleep is absolutely key for this, especially if you want to build in a training program.

If you are reading this and have very young kids that are keeping you awake at night, then I completely empathize with you.

Hard training may be out for the meantime, but trust me, simply becoming hydrated and following some other simple steps will hopefully help you through a difficult period.

Whilst you can't always control how much sleep you get each night (due to the little ones), you now understand that hormones ghrelin and cortisol affect your hunger. Be aware of this and, if nothing else, stay hydrated.

If you are reading this and have poor sleep simply due to staying up late watching Netflix, we can fix this.

Getting the right amount of sleep (and staying hydrated) are the key ingredients for long term health and fat loss success.

You should wake up feeling refreshed in the morning, no matter what age you are.

At forty-two years old, I am living proof of that. This is not to impress you, more to impress upon you that it can be done.

A lot of men tell me they struggle with sleep, but really, they aren't helping themselves. So, let's start with the basics.

Firstly, you want to be going to bed feeling tired, due to the fact that you have actually moved your arse during the day! This could be a simple walk outside for forty-five minutes. It doesn't have to be a strenuous workout.

Secondly, if you are increasing your water intake, then taper off in the early evening. This will avoid you having to get up in the middle of the night to pee! I normally get my two or three litres in before 5pm. Then I just have one Pepsi max in the evening.

Now, this is the hard part and you must give

it time. Unlike getting hydrated, you can't just fix this in an instant. You must be patient with the process.

If you struggle to drop off, then I suggest you have zero television or access to your phone for an hour before bed. Perhaps you could read a book or listen to some relaxing music instead. You could even get some black-out blinds in your bedroom and use earplugs to block out any distracting noises.

I've used earplugs for over twenty years and I absolutely swear by them.

I also love a fan on in the background, whether it's summer or winter, but there's no real need for that – that's just me being weird!

Make your bedroom the place you go to sleep and not a place for digital distractions.

- Make the effort to become more active during the day so that you're actually tired when going to bed.
- Ensure you're hydrated, but have tapered off after 5pm.
- Have your bedroom free from digital distractions so that it's set up for a good night's sleep.

After you can tick off the above, there is also some supplementation we can look at, but the following is pointless unless you are already following the above points.

Before bed, you might want to try a simple 'Night time tea' (available in all health stores or online). I often use the brand called 'Pukka' but there are many different kinds.

This is a nice, simple first step to add into an improved nighttime routine. I would give this a go for a few weeks to see how you get on.

If you are still struggling, then we could look at adding in some ZMA. Zinc and Magnesium is another natural supplement, available from all health stores. It's taken in a capsule form, which has been proven to aid a deeper sleep and help boost testosterone.

Also, you should know that improving the length and quality of your sleep is also the best natural testosterone booster for men.

In fact, if you are over the age of thirty, inactive and consistently suffering with poor sleep, it's highly likely that your testosterone will be plummeting through the floor.

ZMA is cheap, safe and effective. However, it will also give you crazy dreams, just to warn you!

I use ZMA every night to aid my quality of sleep.

You could combine a night time tea with two or three ZMA capsules, forty-five minutes before bed. With a detox of electronics beforehand, this could set you up nicely for an improved sleep within a matter of weeks.

My third recommendation is CBD oil – cannabis oil. It is perfectly legal and available in all health stores or online.

I discovered the sleep aiding benefits of CBD oil when I first purchased some back in 2017. I had chronic hip pain that just wasn't going away, despite lots of stretching and mobility. I bought a brand called 'LOVE CBD' and went for the 800mg strength, which cost around £45.

I started with two sprays under my tongue each evening. It wasn't necessarily the best tasting (I've used a peppermint flavored one ever since), but within just ten days, my hip pain had gone.

Not only this, but I was enjoying extremely deep sleep too!

I have to stress that I was not taking CBD for sleep, nor had I been using ZMA at the time. I gave up taking ZMA when my kids were very young. I thought it was pointless trying to get a deep sleep when my kids were waking me up all the time!

When I tried the CBD, I have to say it gave me a slightly better quality of sleep (in comparison with ZMA) although the crazy dreams from both were on par!

I did however find that it took me a little more time to come around in the morning if I had taken CBD in comparison with ZMA.

Never take the two together!

These days, if I take either (separately), I will always ensure I don't have an early alarm, as I won't get the full benefit of the supplement and wouldn't want to risk feeling groggy in the morning. You really want to ensure you have the time to get the best from it in terms of sleep.

I cannot emphasize enough just how important improved sleep has been in getting me into the shape of my life over the last year.

I will go as far as saying this was THE ULTI-MATE FACTOR.

Even though my sleep improved when my kids got a little older, pre-lockdown I was still being rudely awoken by alarms three to four times a week.

I was extremely busy as an in-person trainer, getting up at 5am (for boot camps and PT) with the alarm always cutting my sleep short.

Don't get me wrong, I adapted. I would sometimes have car naps (my favourite) during the day, but the early and regular alarms often made me feel jaded and hungry.

As a PT, you go where the business is and a LOT of clients wanted to train early before work. As the sole provider for my family, I never turned work down.

However, it did catch up with me.

I remember back in 2019, on my holiday in Turkey, I was sitting by the pool, reflecting.

I was in bits after running in Europe's Toughest Mudder only the week before. I had prepared hard for twelve weeks prior, whilst still getting up very early most days.

As I've already stated, sleep is absolutely necessary for recovery, but I was training hard and not recovering.

I told myself that when I got back home from holiday, I would speak to some of my early morning clients and tell them I was no longer available.

It was a big decision, but quite frankly I was knackered. I was also becoming extremely resentful of the alarm (especially during the winter when it was so cold and dark).

After twelve years in the industry, this was a massive decision. I really worried that I was letting clients down, but of course they understood.

I didn't totally give up my early starts, but I certainly halved them. This really helped, and lying in until 7.45am a few mornings a week was amazing!

Despite not doing as many early starts as I had the previous year, I was still up early a few times a week. I was here, there and everywhere! I was heavily involved in coaching both my kids local football teams. Coupled with weekend live workouts and a very busy PT schedule, I was what I call a 'busy fool'.

My weekends were mental. I was racing from a live workout early on a Saturday morning to teaching boot-camp straight afterwards. Then rushing home for my son's football and rushing back again to take my other son to boxing. You catch the drift! I'm sure many of your lives look the same?

Then BANG! Lockdown came.

Gyms closed. No boot camp. No school run. All in one fell swoop.

It's fair to say, I officially shit myself (as many

self-employed business owners did).

For a few nights, I stayed up late drinking, panicking that I was going to lose everything I had worked for.

One morning, I didn't want to get out of bed.

My missus had a quiet work in my ear. "Come on Tregs, pull it together. You are our motivator. We need you to be upbeat, otherwise we all go down."

She never really needs to give me a pep-talk so I knew how poignant it was.

I immediately tried to pull my head out of my arse. After a discussion with my team, we pivoted hard and went full steam ahead, online.

I no longer had to be anywhere. I didn't need to get up to drive to a gym. I didn't have to rush to get the kids to school. I started to do everything online.

This meant a complete change in schedule.

For the first 12-16 weeks, I was still up early and putting in a shift on live workouts inside our Brotherhood area, which had seen a massive influx in clients.

By around July, my body was battered, but we had added a few hundred extra clients and launched our Inner Circle coaching program.

I was able to hand over the morning live workouts to some amazing coaches, which took the pressure off me.

My business was set up to go in a completely different direction online. By handing over the reins to my other coaches, I was able to really rest and recover.

During this time, I decided that even when things went back to normal, I would no longer go back to the grind like before.

The pandemic had presented me with a unique opportunity to restructure, build my business online, enjoy more family time and have a better connection with my partner. It would also mean that I no longer had to do those grueling early starts!

Fridays would always be my longest day; up at 5am, home at 8pm. I did it for years and just got on with it, because I loved my job. However, I decided this would be no more.

I decided not to do any work past midday on a Friday and I've stuck to that ever since!

Around September 2020, I set myself a challenge. I was going to go ninety days, no booze.

I'd booked a holiday to Turkey for two weeks with the family, but my missus panicked when she saw that it might be added to the quarantine list. She was adamant that the kids shouldn't have any more time off school.

Thankfully I found a loophole and got a full refund.

However, I was so gutted I couldn't go away, especially after the growth of my online business and all the work I'd put in. Instead, I behaved like I'd gone on an all-inclusive – I drank beers every night for two weeks!

My weight went up from around 87kg to 91kg. I thought to myself: *'This is ridiculous!'*

'I'm doing all these live workouts and I don't have to rush around like I was before. My stress levels are lower, my outgoings are drastically reduced and I can get better quality sleep with no alarms. This is a perfect opportunity to level up my physique, in the same way I have done with my business!'

So, I decided to do: ninety days – no booze.

I'd done it in the past with great success prior to a half-marathon, but I'd also tried it in 2019 and failed after forty-five days. I knew it wasn't going to be plain-sailing.

For a start, I was going to have to navigate our first Inner Circle meet-up in Cardiff within a few short weeks of starting. Added to that, it was my birthday in October.

Interestingly, the ninety days of no booze quickly became one hundred days, then one hundred and fifty, then two hundred! I got into the shape of my life and it was easier than anything I'd done in the past.

Why? I was no longer going around tired. I was no longer waking up with a jolt due to continuous early alarms. I was no longer working crazy long hours, surviving on a poor night's sleep, trying to train hard and not recovering.

My sleep regularly started to hit nine hours plus, and I was waking up feeling amazing.

No insane hunger, great energy, improved discipline and never feeling like I 'deserved' a beer because I'd had such a busy day rushing around.

Don't get me wrong, I was still busy working on my online business, but I wasn't a busy fool, chasing my tail and consistently sacrificing sleep and recovery to earn a crust.

The fact that my major focus became a good night's sleep, everything else became easy.

Like I said, if you're tired, you're fucked!

The improved sleep and fact that I wasn't chasing my tail, was the KEY in helping me maintain this level. Throughout Christmas, New Year and many months afterwards, it helped me to get into my finest shape and health at the age of forty-two.

You might be reading this, thinking, 'It's alright for you Tregs. Being able to go online and get a better quality of life'.

I will just say, that when the opportunity was presented, I grabbed it. I took stock and decided to restructure my life. I didn't just sit on my arse. I looked for improvements and my whole world changed.

I can't fix your work. I can't change your shift patterns or stop the kids from waking you up in the middle of the night, but I can make you aware of just how important sleep is.

If reading this chapter makes you think about how you can make some small changes; changes which will lead to improved sleep, then I've done my job.

CHAPTER NINE

Getting started –
Knowing your numbers

OKAY, SO HERE IS WHERE we finally get to the nitty gritty and give you a real understanding of how fat loss occurs.

Remember that I want you to speed up and not slow down. When you lose weight safely, you will not only experience an increase in energy, but your confidence will rocket too!

Whilst there are many psychological factors to consider when it comes to weight loss (that have already been mentioned in this book), it's important to understand how weight loss works.

I've often said that many men fail, but not for the want of trying. It's because they don't understand how weight loss occurs.

Plain and simple; weight loss occurs when you expend more calories through daily movement and exercise, than you consume via food and drink.

Most of you probably knew this anyway, but here's the thing; some of you probably won't know what I'm about to tell you.

You burn calories just by being alive!

That's correct, just existing as a living and breathing organism, burns calories.

How fucking cool is that?

The calories you burn just by being alive is known as your <u>BMR.</u>

Basal Metabolic Rate

Every one of us has a different BASAL META-BOLIC RATE.

My current BMR is 1723 calories.

This is based on me being:–

- Male
- Aged 42
- 5ft 10
- 82kgs

You can work yours out here:
https://www.30plusmensfitness.com/calorie-calculator/

This is why it annoys me when you hear people say things like: "Well if you eat that burger, you'll have to run six miles to burn it off."

Incorrect – you can burn it off just by being alive!

Now, here is the great thing – You will ALWAYS burn more than your BMR!

It gets better, right?

Your BMR is the calories you burn simply by being alive based on your stats – even with zero movement, not even fidgeting!

If you add some daily movement (and even some exercise) to your day, you are going to see that ramp up even more!

So, let's move on to the second thing that contributes to our total daily energy expenditure (TDEE).

It's called N.E.A.T. – Non-Exercise Activity Thermogenesis.

If you've never heard of it, then let me tell you, this is a complete game changer.

This is the number of calories you burn off on a day-to-day basis, just by moving.

Think: walking as the most basic principle. This is why I'm so passionate about setting clients a step goal. Years ago, I would have laughed if I heard myself giving the advice I do now, but the truth is, you can **WALK** your way to weight loss.

Simply moving more consistently each day,

even at a low intensity, can be a huge contributor to overall daily calorie expenditure. And the best thing? Anyone, no matter how out of shape or unfit, can try to move a little more.

It doesn't have to be high intensity training. In fact, for many of you who are just getting started, you really only have to hit more steps!

'What's the catch?' I hear you cry!

No catch! You simply have to find ways to get more steps in!

I always tell clients: 'Get creative with your steps.' It will take some time out of your day and it will require some planning. However, I cannot re-iterate this strongly enough: If you aren't committing to a daily step goal, you are missing the greatest, easiest and most pleasurable way to burn more calories.

Whilst high intensity exercise burns more calories in a shorter period of time, increasing your steps can still illicit a similar response without putting trauma on unconditioned joints and ligaments. This is perfect for heavier guys or those who simply can't bear the idea of going too hard.

The only downside I guess, is that it will take more time.

Each and every one of us will have different levels of N.E.A.T.

If you are on your feet for a living, then you are already in a fantastic position! Sat down all day at a laptop? Like I said, it's time to get creative.

So, let's look at simple ways to ramp up our N.E.A.T:

- Family / Dog walks
- Going to the park with your kids
- Household chores – hoovering, mowing the lawn, hanging up the washing
- Getting involved with your kids' sports or coaching
- Walking to work
- Taking the stairs instead of a lift

You catch my drift!

You might have looked at those things previously and thought they were just a load of hassle. Guess what? I did too! However, once I learned about N.E.A.T, my thought processes changed completely. I'm hoping they do for you too!

Listen, years ago I would have scoffed at a walk. I always felt I had to either 'go hard or go home' in order to lose weight.

Sure, I would go for family walks (often with my kids in buggies), but it would never have been with the same zest and enthusiasm as when I discovered N.E.A.T.

I had been working with an old friend from school (and bodybuilder) called Renzo. I was having some one-to-one sessions with him at the time. I was struggling with the boys being young and lack of sleep. Despite being a PT, I needed a kick up the arse. I tried a different gym, away from my normal environment.

Whilst we would hit the weights, he would always bang on about how I needed to get my steps in. He called it L.I.S.S (Low intensity steady state), but to be honest I would just glaze over.

He would enthuse about how he would walk to and from the gym to ensure he got his steps in.

I asked him what cardio he did to cut down his body fat for shows. He told me it would simply be walking. He said that his job as a postman was perfect for him.

Then, at the start of 2016, I remember having an in-depth conversation with a fellow PT at the gym who was qualified in sports science.

I merely told him I was puzzled by how much weight I'd dropped in the first month of the year.

I hadn't actually been training that much because my coaching schedule was so busy.

He said: "Well, if you're back-to-back coaching all day, your NEAT is sky-high, so that's the reason."

All of a sudden, I paid attention, because it was relevant to me. Everything Renzo had been talking about; all clicked into place right there.

It was true, I hadn't had much time to train because it was January and, like most personal trainers in January, I was run off my feet.

Personal trainers don't sit down and can often put in ten hours a day. That's exactly what I had been doing.

I was now sold on N.E.A.T.

I hope I'm selling it to you too because it was literally game-changing for both my clients and myself.

Now that I was convinced about the success of N.E.A.T, I would jump at the chance to take the kids to the park and pick them up from school on foot.

If the missus asked me to put the hoover on or hang the washing up, I did it with enthusiasm. It was going to up my steps, therefore up my N.E.A.T and contribute to overall daily calorie expenditure!

Now right now as I pen this, I have a daily step goal of 15,000.

Yours doesn't have to be that high, but it needs to be more than what you're currently doing.

So, let's take a look at my average daily calorie burn through my BMR + N.E.A.T (15k steps a day) combined.

BMR = 1723

+ N.E.A.T (15k steps a day) = 600

= 2323 calories

Yep, having a 15k step goal can add a massive 600 calories onto my total daily energy expenditure and we haven't even discussed actual training yet!

Now, 15k steps does take some time and I have to make a very conscious effort to move daily, but remember, this is done leisurely and with ease. So, on a day with no training and just hitting my steps, I can burn 2323 calories a day.

Let's look at the third factor on top of BMR + N.E.A.T: it is called E.A.T

E.A.T has nothing to do with what you put in your gob by the way!

E.A.T stands for:–

EXERCISE

ACTIVITY

THERMOGENESIS

It accounts for the calories burned in planned exercise (basically when you workout). This is really the icing on the fat loss cake!

Just to recap:–

<u>BMR</u> – BASAL METABOLLIC RATE (the calories you burn being alive with no movement whatsoever. You will always burn more than your BMR)

<u>N.E.A.T</u> – NON-EXERCISE ACTIVITY THERMOGENISIS The calories your burn doing daily steps and movement.

<u>E.A.T</u> (EXERCISE ACTIVITY THERMOGENISIS)

The calories you burn working out.

Let's take a look at my workout day to see what my total daily energy expenditure (T.D.E.E) would look like:–

BMR – 1723

N.E.A.T (15k steps) – 600

Workout (kettle bells or run as an example) – 750

Total daily energy expenditure = 3073 (calories burned)

As you can see, that is a pretty decent burn, but let's remember, it's a very active day indeed.

Let's look at a few different variations before we apply all of this to you.

Example 1

Inactive day with minimal N.E.AT and no E.A.T

BMR = 1723

N.E.A.T (less that 5k steps) = 200

E.A.T = 0

Total daily calories expended = 1923

Example 2

An inactive day for N.E.A.T but got a workout in.

BMR = 1723

N.E.A.T (less than 5k steps) = 200

E.A.T = 600

Total daily calories expended = 2523

Example 3

No training but hit my step goal

> BMR = 1723
>
> N.E.A.T (15k steps)= 600
>
> E.A.T = 0

> Total daily calories expended = 2323

Given all of those examples, what is this teaching you?

Basically, the more you move, the more calories you burn.

It's important to remember that you are not always going to be able to train with intensity day in, day out, so keeping up the N.E.A.T on non-training days is key.

You can actually see there's NOT too much difference in:– total daily energy expended on a non-training day with high N.E.A.T, compared with a training day with very little N.E.A.T.

This shows that you don't have to hit the gym with all that high intensity stuff if you're not ready.

High N.E.A.T + E.A.T is the ultimate combo of course, but remember you are NOT going to train hard every day, as you will end up burned out and not recovering.

How can you work out what calories you'll burn with the types of days activities demonstrated above?

Well, you have two options:–

- Using the calculator on our website
- Using a fitness tracker (highly recommended)

I will show you the first one now, but bear in mind, this requires you to be honest with yourself about your level of activity.

Go to: www.30plusmensfitness.com

Select the "calorie calculator" (just like you did when you worked out your B.M.R).

Now use the drop-down menu to select your level of activity (If you are not using a fitness tracker, this may not be entirely accurate). For example, if I wasn't wearing my Garmin, I would input 'moderately active' 3-5 x per week. I believe that would honestly cover my 15k steps a day and 3 to 4 workouts a week.

Let's say you are doing 10k steps daily and maybe 2-3 workouts per week, I would class that as "lightly active".

If you are NOT training and only hitting

around 5k steps a day, I would class that as "sedentary; little or no exercise".

As I have said, if you're not wearing a tracker, you're not going to be getting an entirely accurate reading.

What's the best option? Hands down, it's wearing a fitness tracker. Listen, if you are serious about losing weight and cracking this for the long term, then the best investment you'll ever make is to treat yourself to a decent fitness tracker.

I originally started with Fitbit back in 2016/2017, but I can tell you that they drastically over-calculate your daily expenditure by a whopping 500 calories!

My Fitbit was telling me that I was burning 3000 calories a day, just by doing 12-15k steps and no training! So, of course I ate 3000 calories on those days and guess what? I gained weight!

I ended up actually doing a video called "Don't trust your Fitbit". You can watch it here: https://youtu.be/5aSyYm1xgB8.

So, around 2019, I bought a GARMIN FORE-RUNNER 235 which I still wear and absolutely swear by today!

They retail around £135 – £150, but I got mine for just £50. A client had been gifted an Apple

Watch AND a Garmin Forerunner 235 for her birthday. She wanted to sell the Garmin.

I actually didn't wear it for a while, but finally one day I sat down, charged it up and downloaded the app. I got my head around its features the day before the Cardiff half marathon. I wanted to pace myself and track my 1k times. I was blown away by how great it worked during the race! It gave me my 1k pace throughout and helped me to finish with a cracking time of 1 hour 37 mins.

Don't get me wrong, I had trained hard for the race, but with the help of the Garmin, I was able to track exactly how I was getting on in terms of pace throughout.

After that, I was totally hooked. For a few weeks, I continued to track steps and workouts, quickly realising it was far more accurate than the Fitbit.

In fact, after comparing it with numbers on the calorie calculator, it was pretty much bang-on as accurate as it could be. The scenarios I have given you in this section (about calories burned on different days) are simply what my Garmin has given me. I absolutely swear by it and find it great value. Even though I only paid £50 for it, I would happily pay the full price (ten times over) for giving me an accurate representation of the calories I'm burning.

That's before we even look at sleep! The V.O.2 max, heart rate features and syncing it with the Strava app, make it even more valuable!

Of course, you don't have to go for a Garmin like me. There are even better trackers out there. A lot of my clients rave about the Apple Watch, which looks pretty amazing too. I simply don't have any personal experience of using one.

Honestly, a decent fitness tracker is the absolute KEY if you want to measure your stats accurately. Invest in a decent one and you won't be disappointed.

You may be reading thus far and thinking: 'This all sounds cool, but I'm still not sure <u>WHAT</u> to eat in order to lose weight.'

We have been building to this bit!

I want you to download a FREE app called 'My Fitness Pal'. This is going to help you to track your calories by scanning (or inputting) every bit of food and drink you consume.

Things will start to become much clearer!

I often say: "Spend your calories like you spend your money." Here's how it works:

1lb of fat = 3500 calories.

We tend to look at fat loss on a weekly basis, so let's use the example of creating a deficit of 3500 calories over 7 days. This equates to a 500 deficit a day.

Therefore, you simply need to expend 500 more calories per day via your BMR, N.E.A.T and E.A.T than you take in via food and drink.

Another phrase I often use is: "What gets measured, gets managed."

This could be a real light bulb moment, as you may have never looked at it like this before. Let's use myself as an example.

If I have an active day and burn 2800 calories, yet I only consume 2300 calories, then I will have a 500 deficit.

If have a less active day and burn only 2300 calories, but I only consume 1800, I will still have a 500 deficit.

A deficit is a deficit.

The key to weight loss is to eat less and move more, but remember, you won't always have the chance to exercise.

It's really important to know that exercise isn't the be-all and end-all for fat loss. Of course it helps, but you <u>CAN</u> still lose weight without exercise, simply by eating a little less.

This works both ways. You gain weight by consuming more calories than you expend via your B.M.R, N.E.A.T and E.A.T.

If you're reading this and carrying too much fat, then please remember, it is just stored energy. It's a result of not moving enough for the calories you have been consuming. For example, I could have an active day and burn 2800 calories, but if I eat more than that, I will be in a surplus and gain weight!

Many people assume that by exercising HARD, they have the green light to eat anything, but it simply doesn't work that way!

Why do you think I was an overweight runner? I didn't understand energy balance = calories in – versus – calories out.

There was one time when I ran four half-marathons in a month, yet I ended up gaining weight!

So, now we are clear:– a daily deficit of 500 calories a day, over a period of 7 days, will give you a 3500 deficit for the week. A 3500 deficit will illicit 1lb fat loss a week.

You're probably thinking that all you have to do is go away and create that 500 a day deficit? Easy as that?

Well actually my friend, it gets even better than that.

It might look easy on paper to create a 500 daily deficit. However, it's important to understand that, despite being equipped with this knowledge, you're still going to have days where you feel hungrier than others.

There'll be days (at the weekend for example), when you'll want to eat more than others.

Remember I told you I wanted you to lose that 'on or off the wagon' mentality?

Well, this is where this whole dieting game becomes so much more simplified.

Okay, so here goes:–

Sticking to the magical weekly 3500 deficit as the example, it doesn't matter if you're in deficit by an exact 500 on a daily basis, as long as the goal deficit is achieved at the end of the seven days.

Some days the deficit could be bigger! Maybe you trained hard and did plenty of steps so your TDEE was quite high, yet you simply weren't that hungry.

Other days, the deficit could be less. Maybe you didn't train or hit your steps. Perhaps you felt hungry due to the training you did the day before.

Maybe one day you break even on calories? Maybe one day (God forbid!) you even go over! It doesn't matter, as long as the goal deficit is achieved by day seven!

Can you see how much this is going to set you free?

Can you see why going to bed in a surplus is no longer a fail, a cheat or a treat? You simply went over your calories for the day!

Let's take a look at some examples below:–

Monday – 500 deficit

Tuesday – 250 deficit

Wednesday – 250 deficit

Thursday – 1000 deficit

Friday – 500 deficit

Saturday – 0 deficit (break-even)

Sunday – 1000 deficit

Total weekly deficit = 3500 calories = 1lb
    weight loss

The example above shows a few different deficits during the week and a break-even on Saturday. This means you get to eat more at the weekend – pretty cool right?

Let's look at another one:–

Monday – 1000 deficit

Tuesday – 500 deficit

Wednesday – 500 deficit

Thursday – 750 deficit

Friday – 750 deficit

Saturday – Break even

Sunday – Break even

Total weekly deficit = 3500 calories = 1lb
weight loss

The example above shows a pretty aggressive daily deficit during the week, but then two days of break-even calories at the weekend (which is when we all like to eat more, right?).

Despite the weekend at break-even calories on both days, the 3500 deficit still occurs because of the slightly more aggressive nature of the deficits mid-week.

This a method that I like to use and has been a real eye opener for many clients. It breaks them free from the shackles of conventional dieting because it's so flexible.

This, my friend, is 'flexible dieting' and it's a complete game changer.

Later in this book, I'm going to go into more detail on two methods called:–

- 'calorie borrowing' (partly shown above) and
- 'calorie cycling'

Both make up the 'flexible' approach to dieting that I'm discussing.

However, for now I want to move slightly away from calories, as we have not even looked at what foods to eat yet.

For many of you picking up this book, you may have been expecting some kind of 'diet' plan with a list of foods to eat and those to avoid.

I'm not going to give you that. Years ago I would have, but not now.

Truth be told, back in 2012, the message was all about something called 'clean eating'.

This was very much the buzz term in the industry at the time. It involved a very low carbohydrate diet (cutting out bread, rice and pasta), but eating lots of vegetables and protein (fish, chicken, eggs and meat).

There is absolutely nothing wrong with protein and veggies – in fact it should form the basis of your diet if you want to get leaner. However, this was pretty much ALL that you could eat; even fruit was being demonized at the time because of its sugar content!

If you ate 'clean' for say, a 28-day period, you would drop a shed load of weight, fast.

Unbeknown to me at the time, I was putting clients into a MASSIVE calorie deficit by simply removing so many food groups.

It's extremely important to know that for every 1 gram of carbohydrate you ingest, you store 3 grammes of water. So, when you switch to a very low carb diet, your body also drops a lot of water. This is reflected on the scale. It might sound great, but it's mainly water, not fat!

You may think: 'Okay! Simply cut out all bread, rice and pasta and get lean!' However, this is simply NOT sustainable in the long term. At some point, you're going to 'fall off the wagon'. It's this mentality that we are trying to eradicate!

Clients (myself included) would follow this extremely restrictive way of 'clean eating' for 28 days, only to beg for the end to come.

Often when the plan finished, they would post impressive scale results, but end up on an epic binge afterwards.

A few short weeks later, they would ask: 'Tregs, when is the next plan? I need to get back on the wagon!'

Like I said, this was the same for me too.

I could eat clean for a period of time, only to crash by weekend two or three. I'd end up on an epic binge, which would involve four or five packets of crisps, four or five chocolate bars, and an abundance of bread and cheese.

I used to tell myself it was okay; that it was a 'cheat day' and it was 'boosting my metabolism'. The 'cheat day' was a big 'thing' in the fitness industry at the time too.

I went on paid courses where we were being told to make sure clients ate 'clean' for 28 days. They then went on to instruct that clients would be allowed a cheat day or a cheat meal. This would apparently give the metabolism a 'jolt' and help you burn even more fat!

I'm cringing as I type this, because I actually bought into it!

We introduced 'cheat days' into our program on the second Sunday of the plan and told clients it was a green light to eat whatever they wanted – just no booze!

I'd get reports of guys going on epic all-day binges, starting with chocolate for breakfast, Domino pizza with all the extras, then loads of sweets.

Most men were consuming between 4000-5000

on those cheat days, but then posting about how awful they felt afterwards.

Not only this, but many clients found it hard to 'get back on the clean eating wagon' the next day. They often felt like they wanted to continue eating the crap we'd permitted them to eat the day before.

I decided that a 'cheat day' was too much and started to replace it with a 'cheat meal'. At least there would be some boundaries, but even this didn't sit well with me. The 'clean eating' message was still too restrictive and it started to bother me.

Like I said earlier, pre-kids, I found it easy to eat 'clean'. Even with epic fortnightly weekend binges, I was able to stay lean because there wasn't any real stress in my life. I could adhere to living off meat and veggies for ninety percent of the time.

However, once the kids came along, it all went horribly wrong. Trying to eat a restrictive diet when you're knackered, just added more stress to my life. The binges became all too often and I gained two stone in 2015.

It was around the time that I started to see Steven the counsellor. I was growing an awesome business, but unable to stick to the message I was promoting. Thankfully, I also discovered 'flexible dieting'.

The message from the 'flexible dieting' camp, was that you can eat all your favorite foods (pizza, ice cream, chocolate, crisps) and even drink alcohol, but in moderation!

The goal was to simply make those calories fit into your daily target (see why I've shown you how to work out your numbers?)

To be honest, I couldn't get my head around it at first.

My mind-set was 'How can someone eat pizza and stay lean?

Also, how can you eat only a few slices? Surely once you've started eating pizza, you've ruined your diet, so you might as well just go ahead and eat the whole thing!

I actually mocked 'flexible dieters' at first, but there I was, unable to stick to clean eating, two stone heavier, restricting foods, then binging.

After one of my first sessions with the counsellor, he told me to go away and just eat one packet of crisps or one bar of chocolate.

He told me that labeling food 'good' or 'bad' was a major part of my problem.

It blew my mind!

I was so caught up in this mind-set of: if it's not meat, fish or veggies, then it's not clean!

It had got to the point where I was limiting fruit because of the (natural) sugar content. I was even scared to chew gum because I was worried it would set off an insulin spike, which would put me into fat storage mode!

Honestly the fitness industry and the message at the time has so much to answer for. It was literally creating dis-ordered eating for both coaches and clients!

A combination of the following things set me off on a new journey; seeing a counsellor for help with poor eating habits, learning about 'flexible dieting', using the new buzzword N.E.A.T, and fitness trackers to help me track steps.

I remember downloading 'My Fitness Pal' and thinking; *'Okay, I'll track my calories, try out this deficit thing and eat some 'unclean foods', but there's no way this will work'.*

Even though I was failing at 'clean eating', I was still convinced that sticking to it was the only way!

I allowed myself 1800-2000 calories for the day. I wasn't obsessed with a massive deficit because I wasn't convinced that this new plan would work.

I thought to myself; *'Okay, I'll have that packet of crisps. I'll let myself eat that chocolate bar – and I'll pick my favorite ones too!'*

I ate my favorite packet of crisps (Salt and Vinegar discos). At 34 grammes, they are only 181 calories! *'Not too bad!'* I thought. I can enjoy them and it barely makes a dent in my daily intake.

What about my favorite chocolate bar? Let's look at a Cadburys whole nut; it's around 250 calories.

How about a Fruit Pastille lolly? I couldn't believe this was just 60 calories! I'd be able to enjoy one in the summer without thinking I'd ruined my diet.

At the time, I really enjoyed drinking Guinness, so I checked out the calories. I was actually pleasantly surprised to learn that a pint of the black stuff had only 210 calories! I presumed it would be around 400!

I have to say, this 'change' did not happen overnight. There was a lot of resistance to it. After all, I was a fitness coach promoting 'clean eating' and making good money online. However, learning about calories was a massive eye opener and as time went on, I started to treat my calories like money.

I would tell myself I had a certain amount of calories (money) to 'spend' every day and once I ran out, that was simply it.

I could stop eating (spending) or I could carry on eating and go into my overdraft (essentially a calorie surplus and fat gain).

It was a revelation.

I started to drop fat and get leaner using this new, more sustainable method. Being able to factor in my favorite 'junk' foods and the odd alcoholic beverage along the way was liberating.

I was flabbergasted (in a good way) that I could still drink alcohol and lose weight. I had previously told myself that if I had a drink, I was off the wagon.

Around that time, I recorded a podcast with guy I have a lot of respect for – Phil Learney. Whilst talking about 'flexible dieting', I mentioned the term 'junk food'. Phil immediately interrupted and said; "Tregs! Don't call it junk food! Call it 'slightly less nourishing, higher calorie food'. He went on to say that this would create a better relationship with food by simply not labeling it as 'bad'.

He told me: "When you eat slightly less nourishing, higher calorie food, understand that you are simply using up more calories for less nutrition."

You can still eat those foods, but they won't fill you up or keep you satisfied for as long. More nourishing (and less calorie) foods will keep you going longer.

This compounded everything for me. I was sold on the idea.

The counselling (which lasted around eight months), combined with discovering flexible dieting, had opened up a whole new world for me. After almost ten years in the fitness industry, I felt liberated.

I noticed how my binges had disappeared. Giving myself permission to have the occasional packet of crisps and the odd chocolate bar had satisfied the craving, preventing the urge to binge.

Because I was no longer telling myself I couldn't have these foods, I no longer yearned for them. It actually turned me into a 'cleaner' eater. 'Cleaner eater' – now I hate that term, but what I mean, is that I was actually able to sustain a healthier diet consistently. I no longer felt the urge to go off on crazy binges.

My counselling sessions were coming to an end and my new system of tracking calories was really helping me. Added to that, my boys were now 3-4 years old and were finally starting to sleep through the night.

I felt re-born.

It was as though a huge weight had been lifted. I had a clear vision of how I wanted to move forward.

However, there was one problem.

I now had to come out and tell my large following and client base, that I had found a new way.

The fitness industry had been going in this direction for a while and I had been talking about 'calories in vs. calories out' in my member's area. However, now I needed to tell the general public.

I always tried to do things with integrity. I only wanted the best for my clients.

There's a fantastic quote: "You only know what you know". This couldn't have rung any truer for me.

I recorded a podcast simply titled; "I was wrong". I explained everything that I had learned. Thankfully, it was very well received.

From that point on, we started to tweak our program and offer the option of tracking calories.

Yes, there was some resistance from clients at first, just as I had felt personally. However, it was down to me to re-train clients' thought processes and educate them. It was my duty of care to teach this new way so that they never felt 'on or off' the wagon again.

We gave clients two options; one, was to stick with the previous 'clean eating', but aim for a less restrictive approach, and the second, was to track calories.

Even with my updated message, I want you to know that you don't have to track your calories initially, if you're completely new to this game.

Of course, at some point, you're going to need to track your calories. However, if you're reading this book and perhaps you would deem yourself to be quite overweight, then understand that you don't need to track your calories initially.

Perhaps you're returning from injury. Maybe you've gained a lot of weight since the kids were born. Perhaps you've just been lazy for a few years. There's a simple way to get started before you even think of downloading a fitness tracker.

1) Up the steps

If a 'heavier' client comes to me, I will just encourage them to move more initially. Like I've already said, N.E.A.T is key. Heavier clients will find it easier to simply up their steps rather than start hard training.

How many steps a day? That is entirely down to you. Don't set an unrealistic step goal. You'll only end up not being able to reach it and then feel demoralized. Set the bar low enough and go from there.

I recently worked with a client who had no idea how many steps he was doing. After the pandemic hit, he knew he was moving less. There was no commute to the office and he was working from home. He guessed he was doing around 3500-4000 steps per day.

I told him to purchase a Garmin so that we could measure accurately. I then set him a realistic target of between 5k and 7k steps per day. I told him to do no less that 5k steps, and no more than 7k, so that the seven-day target was between 35k-49k.

He quickly became accustomed to that, no problem. A few weeks later, we revisited it and increased it to a 6k-8k target per day. He got fitter, lost weight and became more confident. The more he became used to each target, we were able to keep increasing the goal.

When we finished our three months of sessions together, he was achieving upwards of 12k steps a day. It really helped his overall daily calorie expenditure and mental health!

2) Eat more greens

We all know vegetables are great for us, right? But why exactly is this?

Well, not only do they contain lots of vitamins and minerals, but they're water based, which means that they expand in your stomach. They're going to help you feel fuller, for longer.

Think: Super-nourishing, filling, very little calories!

By replacing your plate of pasta with a plate of veggies, it's going to save you a shed-load of calories, and leave you feeling fuller for longer.

3) Get protein on the plate

Think: Meat, fish, eggs.

Not only is protein essential for muscle repair, it is also satiating enough to make you not want to binge on it.

Whilst carbohydrate (bread, rice, pasta) and protein have the same number of calories per gramme, carbs get the bad rep. Why? Because it's very easy to over-eat carbs!

Think about the last time you binged on cakes. Now, compare that to the last time you binged on chicken.

My guess is that you have never binged on chicken, right?

Not only does protein help keep you fuller for longer, but it also creates what we call a T.E.F (Thermic effect of food).

Because it's the hardest food for the body to digest, the body can ramp up its metabolism to help with digestion. This may only be a minor thing, but if you start to eat more protein as part of an improved lifestyle, this will also play a positive part.

A fitness guru I follow in the States, always says: P+V first.

Protein and veggies first.

If you fill your plate with protein and veggies first, you'll not go wrong. Ultimately, you'll feel more satisfied and nourished, for less calories.

4) Reduce 'slightly less nourishing' higher calorie food (remember we don't call it 'junk' any more)

Perhaps you are someone who enjoys 4-5 takeaways per week. Whilst it may not be healthy, the days of me telling you to completely cut that out, are gone.

I would merely ask you to halve that initially, in order to lose weight. This is something that many fail to consider. Lots of new clients believe they have to completely change everything in one go. We have already established; this can be dangerous.

5) Hydrate and sleep

As I've already explained, these are the ultimate factors and by getting these right, it will ensure your satiety. It will also help your focus to remain intact, which in turn, helps you to follow the other pointers.

CHAPTER TEN

Mastering your weekends – calorie borrowing

There is NO WAGON!

I HOPE THAT YOU ARE NOW starting to see that there is NO wagon!

I continually tell clients: "You are either over or under your calorie allowance for the day."

You do NOT have to crash, burn and binge, simply because you had a higher calorie day mid-week!

As per the examples I gave earlier, you can actually use your calorie allowance over a seven-day period, rather than going day-by-day.

You go over one day? No problem, you simply pull it back the next.

This actually sets you free and liberates you from the shackles of conventional dieting.

You have a few mid-week beers and a takeout? No problem.

Remove the guilt.

Simply wake up the next day, get hydrated, maybe skip breakfast, up your steps, slightly reduce starchy carbs and up the veggies. Maybe do a workout, but don't view it as a punishment.

You don't have to go mad; just pull those numbers back in.

This takes away the feeling of failure. It also helps you to break free from that 'I'll start again on Monday' mentality.

We no longer have to have that attitude of: 'all bets are off'. Nor do we have to write the week off, just because one day had higher calories than the others. We simply play the numbers game.

Remember, one 'bad' day (or higher calorie day) won't make you fat. It's the reaction to that belief, and the subsequent four-day binge afterwards, that will make you gain fat.

I was that guy.

It happened far too much when my kids were young. It was awful and I hated it. That's when I decided 'enough was enough' and got help.

I'm so happy and grateful that I've found a new way; a way that I can show you. The 'on/off wagon' mentality was ruining my life, and I'm guessing it may be doing the same for you.

I want to take a look at the weekend, because

let's face it, when we're trying to get fit (and/or lose fat), the weekends can be the most difficult.

It's as if we're programmed to reward ourselves with takeaways and alcohol, because of the long week we've had. Combine that with the old 'relax and put your feet up' mentality, and it's easy to see why the weekend can become our 'weak-end'. We end up going into Monday feeling tired, lethargic and starting all over again.

Believe me, I have been that guy, time and time again. Yes, even as a personal trainer – both before, and after, the kids came along.

Between 2014 and 2016, before my counseling and before I discovered flexible dieting, my relationship with food was at an all-time low.

Often, after a long week of coaching, I would reward myself with all of my 'banned' foods. Splurging on things like pizza, crisps, and chocolate, I would tell myself it was a 'cheat' weekend and I'd be back on form on Monday.

Looking back now, I can see how dis-ordered this was.

Having said that, pre-kids and with minimal stress, it WAS always easy to 'get back on it'. By training hard and eating 'clean' (I fucking hate that term now) during the week, I always seemed to maintain my weight.

Fast forward to: kids coming along, regular hospital visits for the boys, the upkeep of a big house, staff to manage, no sleep and a constant stream of shitty nappies, it wasn't so easy.

My weekend food behaviors actually got a LOT worse.

When I say that this went on ALL weekend, I mean it went on ALL weekend – even into Sunday night!

Often on a Sunday, I'd wake up very groggy and start the day with one or two bowls of cereal. Then a big roast and a few beers, followed by a shed load of cheese and crackers.

Looking back, Sundays could have easily been a 4k – 5k calorie day – and that was on top of the excesses of Friday and Saturday night!

Back then, I had a full-time coach working for me. He always looked after the Monday morning clients, which meant I never had to go in early.

This sounds like a dream, but for me, not having to get up early on a Monday was just a license to carry on eating and drinking.

It was during these times that our sleep was severely broken. I knew that by over-consuming, I was only going to feel doubly worse when the boys woke us in the middle of the night. However, I can see now that it was a form of escapism.

On Mondays, I would feel like absolute garbage; full of remorse, but determined to go 'clean' again and train myself to death in the gym.

Thankfully, I ended up getting the help I needed, but my God, I wish I'd know then what I know now.

If only I'd known about calories, calorie borrowing and the power of N.E.A.T, but I didn't. I guess the lessons learned were all part of my journey.

Look, who doesn't want to enjoy more food on the weekend?

I know I do.

These days, I enjoy lots of lovely food on the weekend, but I am simply more calorie aware rather than an 'all bets are off' approach.

Most of you that are reading this probably have kids. When you have kids, you often find yourself going out for ice cream or a burger at the weekend. You can still do this and you can eat more on the weekends – you just have to move more!

It's as simple as that.

Most guys get to the weekend and think that

it's 'feet-up' time. They tell themselves they can relax and eat all around them! This is the WRONG approach.

The weekend has to become a time to move more and if you have kids, it's the perfect opportunity! Stop putting off going to the park with the kids! Get active with them at the weekend. Not only are they going to love you, but you are also going to love the extra calories burned.

When the kids were very young, we didn't do much exercise all weekend. Sure, we would get out for walks and push them in a pram, but never with the zest I have now!

When they got a bit older and started to sleep through the night, I decided I wanted to try and get back to my best shape. Equipped with my new-found knowledge, and having had eight months of counselling, I told myself I'd 'make the comeback stronger'.

However, I'd addressed that the weekends could still be a danger for me, and I'd need some kind of accountability to prevent me from over-eating and over-boozing.

Initially, I committed to meeting my great friend (and fellow 30+ coach) Brian, on a Sunday morning to train in the gym. We would meet at around 8.30am, which would ensure I'd get to bed at a decent time. It was also the difference between three beers or ten beers!

This worked out really well as I didn't want to let Brian down. It also meant that I was no longer hung-over on a Sunday morning, starving and having to polish off a few bowls of cereal for breakfast!

The simple commitment was probably saving me around 1500-2000 calories between Saturday night and Sunday morning.

With the kids now sleeping through the night, I decided I wanted to notch it up a level.

So, back in 2017, I began doing early morning Saturday workouts on Facebook Live.

I knew this would not only help to grow my business, but it would also give me extra personal accountability. I certainly didn't want to lead a live workout on a hangover! As the face of the business, I wanted to feel and look clear-headed.

I want to wake up feeling great! I want to be able to perform!

That was the motivation driving me.

When I got home on a Friday night, instead of cracking open the booze, I was focused on the live workout the following morning. I spent the time building a buzz on my social media platforms and encouraging others to join in.

This worked like a dream.

I would pencil in a workout during the week, maybe have a gym session, and then get to bed early on a Friday night. The fact that it was a booze free evening saved a good few calories in the process too!

I'd get up feeling fresh, do my live workout session, and be buzzing with endorphins. After that, I would head out to take my boot camp.

Because I was no longer tired and groggy, the afternoon hunger was curtailed. Bakery visits on the way home were a thing of the past!

That's when I decided to do a live workout on a Sunday morning too!

I ran it by my business partner who warned me not to commit to anything I couldn't maintain.

However, I was really feeling the benefits – getting back into shape as well as growing my brand with extra exposure.

I decided I'd go for it.

This totally reshaped my weekend. The focus was performing on camera and bringing energy to the viewers. That meant laying off the booze and enjoying a great night's sleep.

I ended up getting back in shape and loved the excitement of going live every weekend.

Then things went up another level!

I was approached to get involved with my kids' football teams!

The boys had both started playing at mini level and I was always an enthusiastic watcher from the sidelines. When a few of the coaches found out what I did for a living, they advised I should get my FAW coaching badge. They suggested I become involved, telling me I'd be great with the kids. They then went on to list all the benefits of coaching, such as being on the pitch-side, my kids being included in matches and getting involved in their hobby.

I quickly got my qualification and was thrown in at the deep end. I began coaching the under 5's on a Sunday morning!

My weekends looked like this:–

Saturday morning
- Live workout
- Boot camp

Sunday morning
- Live workout
- Kids' football coaching

I would finish my Sunday morning session buzzing with endorphins, before rushing off to coach about thirty kids! It was hard work but I bloody loved it!

I was busy doing something I loved, on my feet constantly and my step count went through the roof!

All of a sudden, I had turned my weekends around by becoming committed and accountable. On top of that, my danger areas had been taken care of.

Rather than dragging myself into Mondays feeling overweight and lethargic, I was bouncing into them, full of energy. I had either gotten leaner or maintained my weight over the weekend!

This completely and utterly changed my life. As I write this in 2021, I am still as busy and committed at the weekends. I'm also happier and fitter than ever!

So, I want you to take a look at your danger areas. Is it the weekend? Is that your weak-end? If so, then you may need to do something to secure them.

It might be that you meet somebody for a run on a Sunday or you might go and play tennis.

Whatever it is, it must be something you enjoy and something which will keep you accountable.

It has to excite you in order to give you that level of commitment on the weekend. I don't want you to view it as a punishment; I want you to view it as pleasure.

My weekend live workouts and coaching the kids' footy is ultimate pleasure for me and it serves to keep me lean and active.

Don't get me wrong, I still enjoy a LOT of good grub at the weekend, but these days (with my awareness of calories and calorie borrowing), I can pull it off and still wake up leaner on a Monday.

For instance, lately on a Saturday night (especially during the winter lockdown), the missus and I have been having an Indian takeaway. I save myself around 2000 calories to enjoy a takeaway on a Saturday night.

I think by now you can probably guess how I do this?

Saturday
- Live kettle bell workout at 8.30am (I never eat beforehand). This can burn up to 750 calories easily.
- I'll then have a protein shake with a

banana and some berries around midday.

- In the afternoon, I'll head out for a walk with my partner and our dog. I usually end up completing 15k steps by the time we get home.

- By the time 6pm comes and we order our food, I've built up a massive deficit. I can sit down and enjoy it all guilt-free. I often go to bed still in a slight deficit or at least break even on my calories.

Sunday

My dad (who has lived with us for a few years) makes an amazing roast. Regular as clockwork, he puts it on the table at 1.30pm.

I budget my dad's roast as being around 2000 calories (that gives me flexibility to finish off my son's leftovers too!) FYI, I don't factor in every roast potato to My Fitness Pal. Some of it is guess-work. If I overestimate the roast by a few hundred calories then so be it, but I'm happy with my 2000 cals prediction.

I get up on a Sunday and do another live workout. Sometimes it's two sessions (one for my ladies group too). Okay it's a tad excessive but it's only once a week!

By the time I'm done at 11am, I'm in a massive deficit with a decent step count too (again I never eat before a workout).

I then do a little bit of work, and by the time I've showered and sat down for lunch at 1.30pm, I'm starving!

I really savour the roast, enjoying the fact that I don't have to say 'no' to Yorkshire puddings, and 'allowing' myself to eat roast potatoes, unlike previous times in the past!

I then finish up the day with another protein shake and berries in the evening, coming in at around 2500 cals for the day, but still in a deficit!

So that's how I do it! Still enjoying plenty of lovely food, but moving more and borrowing calories here and there to make my weekend meals fit.

You don't have to swing kettle bells with me, but you do need to make the weekend active.

As I have taught you, this fat loss is a calorie game, so learn how to make them fit for you and break free from the wagon!

CHAPTER ELEVEN

Nutrition for performance – calorie cycling

IF CALORIE BORROWING CAN SET you free on the weekend and help you lose fat, then you're going to love calorie cycling.

If you really enjoy your training, but still want to drop body-fat (like me), this will help take you to the next level. If you want to train hard, then you MUST fuel the performance.

Over the years, when playing around with different diets, I have had some terrible experiences whilst trying to train. I remember trying to go for a run on extremely low calories after a few days of zero carbohydrates. It was not a pleasurable experience! Zero energy, lightheadedness and no leg strength were just a few of the things I experienced.

You see, many people think they have to train hard as well as eat very low calories or low carbs, but this is a recipe for disaster.

A small percentage of people say they perform better on low carbs, but it's highly likely they have upped their fats. For many of you reading this, let's keep it simple.

Carbohydrates are your body's primary energy source; they also keep your brain happy, because the brain is the most glucose-hungry organ in the body.

If you go out for a run or do a cross-fit class, but you've had very low calories, you're going to run out of gas. Just like a car would run out of fuel on a long drive, you need to stop and fill up!

For me, there's no greater feeling that having loads in the tank when you train hard. I train for my mental health, just as much as my physical health. Therefore, it's important to me that I fuel that session to get the most out of it.

If you try to train hard with very little fuel on board, it won't create the output you're looking for. More than likely, you'll have to stop.

When you're sufficiently fuelled, you'll be able to achieve a greater intensity and therefore create a bigger calorie output!

How can we get this balance right? We want to fuel up and enjoy our training, whilst still dropping fat.

Here's how!

I want to tell you about something I got into (for about 12 weeks) that really worked for me over lockdown. It helped me to get lighter and leaner, whilst still pushing very hard in training and also recovering well.

The gyms were closed so I decided I would increase my running. I loved the tranquility of being out on my own and listening to my tunes, which also really helped my mental health.

I started to run on Monday, Wednesday and Friday, anywhere between 12k and 15k. Tuesdays and Thursdays were strict rest days.

On a Saturday and Sunday, I would do my live kettle bell workouts. This was the norm for a good couple of months.

It's kind of the norm that on rest days, you should reduce your calories. However, I started to do something a little unconventional. Remember when you train hard, hunger will always follow you around!

So, I started to go over my calories on Tuesday and Thursdays, sometimes with an 800-calorie surplus! What I found, was that the following day on my runs, I would be flying through them! I was getting some really solid intensity.

I never eat before I run, and my runs were always mid-morning. That means I was in what you could call 'a fasted state', but bear in mind, my body was heavily fuelled from the day before.

Because of both the distance and the intensity, I was creating a massive calorie burn on my runs, of between 1300-1800 calories.

You may be thinking: *'He's just running to burn off the calories he ate the night before. What's the point? Just don't over-eat and don't run!'*

Well yes, you could do that! I've already explained that you don't need to exercise hard to lose fat – it's a calorie game. However, that would be missing the point. The point is, I love running and I love training hard, for so many different reasons.

On the days I was running hard, I didn't eat beforehand. I ran mid-morning and was never hungry immediately after. All I wanted to do straight afterwards, was sit in a hot bath with a cold Pepsi Max (zero calories)!

By the time I did get hungry, it was already mid-afternoon. By then, I'd already hit my step goal, created a great burn from training and was in a massive calorie deficit! I would eat only two meals that day and end up, not only in a big deficit, but also having pulled the surplus back from the day before.

I would then 'tactically' (and guilt-free), increase my calories on my rest day and repeat the process again on the following day's run.

As I used 'calorie borrowing' on the weekend, I would often be in a deficit or at least, break-even. By the end of seven days, I would have achieved my goal deficit of between 0.5 and 1lb of fat loss per week; all by cycling my calories around my training.

This was done with three days in a deficit, two days in surplus and two days break even.

Let me show you how below:–

Sunday (Training day / kettle bells)
Cals in = 2500; Cals out = 3250; Deficit = 750

Monday (15k run)
Cals in = 2200; Cals out = 3300; Deficit = 1100

Tuesday (Rest day)
Cals in = 3000; Cals out = 2200; **Surplus = 800**

Wednesday (15k run)
Cals in = 2200; Cals out = 3300; Deficit = 1100

Thursday (Rest day)

Cals in = 3000; Cals out = 2200; **Surplus = 800**

Friday (15k run)

Cals in = 2200; Cals out = 3300; Deficit = 1100

Saturday (Training day / kettlebells)

Cals in = 2750; Cals out = 3050; Deficit = 300

Total weekly deficit = **2750** (which equates to about 2/3rds of 1lb)

If, like me, you love training hard and want to maximize your performance, then consider calorie cycling!

CHAPTER TWELVE

Intermittent fasting –
The good, the bad and the ugly

I CANNOT WRITE THIS BOOK without including a chapter on Intermittent Fasting. Intermittent fasting (or **'IF'**) has gotten mixed reviews in the industry. It's something that I read about back in 2012. I came across a guy called Brad Pilon who had written a book called 'Eat, Stop, Eat'.

It was the first time I'd heard about intermittent fasting. In a nutshell, it's simply going for a period of time without food.

Hardly rocket science, right?

However, the simple practice can set you free from the shackles of conventional dieting. The most basic common practice is called 16-8, which means you fast for 16 hours and eat your food in an 8-hour window. A simple example would be eating from midday until 8pm and then not eating before or after those hours.

Why would you do this?

Well, in Pilon's book, it evangelized about '**IF**' being able to:

- boost testosterone
- increase metabolism
- clear out toxins from your blood stream
- re-boot an immune system
- help you drop fat!

Of course, I became invested! I started to build intermittent fasting into my online programs from 2013, listing all the reasons I had read about in the book.

I got decent results from it and so did my clients. Simply, it was making us eat less, which (unbeknown to me at the time) was putting us into the magical calorie deficit.

As the years went by and I got older and wiser, I read more up on it. I thought, this all sounds great; 'boost your metabolism, boost testosterone, help with your immune system', but how much of it is true? Do we have any indication of how accurate such claims are?

As I started to learn more about calories-in and calories-out, I thought, let's look at this with a more black-and-white, pragmatic view.

Intermittent fasting can help people reduce the number of daily calories they are eating, simply by excluding a meal. Therefore, it immediately puts them into a deficit.

The way this worked for me (as someone who has openly struggled with his weight over the years) was initially by skipping breakfast.

You see, as a guy who likes big portions, eating three meals a day (no matter how healthy) would put me into a calorie surplus, therefore not aiding weight loss.

You might be reading this, thinking that breakfast is the most important meal of the day; that you need it to boost metabolism. Well guess what? So did I!

Back in 2006, when I studied my personal training diploma, the motto was:

"Eat like a king at breakfast, a prince at lunchtime and a pauper in the evening!"

This is very outdated information, but I believed it because I had paid for the training!

When I started my Boot camps in 2010, I was up at 5am twice a week. I was cooking a six-egg omelette in coconut oil at 5.15am. I didn't even want it because I wasn't hungry! However, I really believed this would 'rev up' my metabolism and help me to lose body fat.

It couldn't have been further from the truth.

What I was actually doing, was having 600 calories that I didn't need or want, just for the sake of speeding up my metabolism!

I learned that breakfast was just to "break-a-fast" and it didn't matter what time of the day you had it. That really set me free.

Most days, I don't get hungry until 10am or 11am. By eating later in the day, it gives me more calories to play with.

I often say: "Choose your hunger".

Why? Well, when you're trying to lose weight, you are giving your body less calories than it needs. Therefore, it uses up stored body fat as energy, resulting in fat loss.

You're going to experience a little bit of hunger when dieting from time to time.

It's key to remember that hunger is okay from time to time – in fact everyone should get in touch with their hunger.

A little hunger can keep you sharp and alert.

What we don't want is "hanger"; hunger and anger combined. This happens when we aggressively diet.

Ask yourself:

When can I tolerate a little hunger?

Personally, I can manage my hunger a lot better in the morning.

Quite often, I'm up, rushing to get the kids to school and then going on to the gym. All I can think about is having a coffee and some water. I'm fine until about 11am and then my body starts to tell me to eat!

Contrary to popular myth, your body is not going to go into 'starvation mode'. It's not going to hold onto body fat when you don't eat breakfast first thing. (Don't worry I once believed that too!)

Why? Well, you've got body fat (just like me); stored energy which will fuel your body.

Prolonging the time you have breakfast will help you to create a calorie deficit, because you'll start eating later in the day.

I prefer to eat more calories in the afternoon. I enjoy my biggest meal in the evening because going to bed with a fuller belly (within reason) helps me to sleep better.

This CAN include carbs after 6pm (and just before bed). If you are in a calorie deficit, you will NOT gain body fat!

Yep, I know, another complete turn-around on what I was once taught. Let me tell you, it's another revelation that can set you free!

Carbohydrate before bed has been proven to aid a better night's sleep, due to the fact that it helps to release a hormone called melatonin.

I have played around with many forms of 'IF', including not eating after 6pm. However, going to bed hungry really affected my sleep and made me tired the next day. We already know just how important a good night's sleep is, in order to keep that nasty hunger hormone ghrelin at bay.

By the way, you don't have to NOT eat breakfast, you don't even have to use 'IF'. Just remember, it's simply a tool you can use to create a calorie deficit, if you so wish.

In my personal experience, I found that when using 'IF' (sensibly), I experienced an increase in energy and concentration. When I say sensibly, I mean fasting for between 16-20 hours.

That little bit of hunger makes me sharper, and as long as I'm sufficiently hydrated, my focus and productivity are high.

I have tried 24-hour fasts, 36-hour fasts and even a 60-hour fast! All for the sake of investigating how it feels, so that I can pass on my experiences to clients.

Back in 2018, I was playing around a lot with 24–26-hour fasts, starting on a Sunday night and fasting until Monday night. Whilst they did get me lean, I wasn't able to train hard.

I love training hard, not only for the physical benefits, but for the mental side of things too. This was something I couldn't do during extended fasts.

On a 24-hour fast, I would often experience an insane surge in energy around the 20-hour mark and feel amazing. I would always ensure I was busy coaching and fully hydrated when doing these long fasts. Don't fast when you're not busy – all you'll think about is food!

When doing a 36-hour fast, it would be extremely difficult to bypass the kitchen and go to bed without food at the end of the day. This would often lead to a disrupted night sleep.

Despite waking up and feeling super lean, the tiredness would soon catch up with me during the day. Upon breaking the fast, I would find it hard to stop eating!

Remember, it's no good fasting if you end up gorging on loads of food afterwards. It'll only put you back into a surplus!

This brings me on to my attempt at a 60-hour fast.

I had joined a group on Facebook that was promoting all the usual hype around fasting. Whilst I wasn't convinced, I was keen to give it a go, especially with the support of the group.

I managed to get to the 44-hour mark. I was in the gym with a client and felt completely drained of energy. I had to sit down, and by the way, there's an unwritten rule that coaches do NOT sit down when training!

All I could think about was food and what I was going to buy straight after the session. I told myself that 44 hours was a massive achievement and that I'd head to the local Subway shop and get a large salad.

I scoffed the salad in no time, and then, without any thought, I immediately went back up and ordered a foot long sub, followed by crisps and chocolate.

I couldn't stop!

Remember what I told you about the psychological effects of going too "aggressive"?

Remember how I told you about my issues with food?

This extended fast brought out all the bad

habits in me and I must have consumed about 4000 calories in one sitting.

It literally wrote off the whole fast and was a big warning to never try to push it that far again.

If you have a poor relationship with food, then a long, drawn-out intermittent fast is not for you.

Anything that is going to test your willpower and make you HANGRY in the long run is not for you.

If you simply want to create a calorie deficit however, skipping breakfast is the easiest way to employ intermittent fasting into your life.

As you know, at weekends, I 'borrow' calories to enjoy a Saturday night curry with the missus and my dad's massive Sunday roast. I simply skip breakfast or lunch to allow me to do that.

Therefore, intermittent fasting doesn't have any magical properties. It is simply one way of creating a calorie deficit.

Should you do it? That my friend, with the benefit of reading this chapter, is entirely down to you.

CHAPTER THIRTEEN

Motivation, goals and habits

A SUBJECT I DISCUSS A LOT is motivation. If you haven't trained with me before, then the following might come as a surprise to you. I truly believe that you must STOP relying on motivation to transform your body, improve fitness and change your life.

Hear me out!

As I say, time and time again, motivation WILL play a part – and that part is merely to get you started.

When the emotional (and physical) pain of gaining weight gets too much, it is often the kick-start we need to decide to change.

There are two types of pain:–

1/ The pain that someone is currently in (For example, unhappy with their weight and consumed by negative self-talk)

2/ The pain of change. Change can be daunting too! Change requires action, commitment and patience.

So, when someone finally becomes sick of how they look, they decide to opt for the pain of change.

You tell yourself: "This is it! I'm going to change! I'm finally going to do something about my body and my fitness!"

Stewing over hurtful comments from people about your weight, you might say to yourself: "I'll show them! I'll prove them wrong this time!"

So, on Sunday night, you prep your food and lay out your gym kit, ready for the next day.

You get through the day, eating well and completing the gym session. You go to bed really happy with yourself.

Then during the rest of the week, this thing called LIFE happens.

You might have a sleepless night with young kids needing attention, your boss might be giving you grief at work, you might even receive an unexpected bill in the post.

These are just a few examples of how life can unfold.

This can lead to missed gym sessions, a day of

poor nutrition, stress and tiredness.

The motivation that you had on Sunday night, the eve of embarking on your new plan, has been sucked out of you by Friday.

Your goal is now a distant memory and all you can think about is downing a few beers and treating yourself to a takeaway. It's like a reward for what the week has thrown at you.

We are humans, and therefore emotive creatures. We seek comfort in excess food and alcohol, reverting back to the habits that caused our weight gain.

It's easily done and it's the reason why most people are caught in a perpetual cycle of starting, stumbling, stopping and sabotaging. Then starting again week after week.

If motivation runs out as quickly as I have highlighted, then what's the answer?

The answer lies in both goals and habits.

Let's look at goals first:

The older I get, (forty-two years old at the time of writing), the more obsessed I become about having goals. Not having a goal literally scares the shit out of me.

I read a quote recently which said: *"Mankind is*

at its happiest when working towards a goal."

I wholeheartedly agree.

For me, it's not just about 'achieving a goal' that excites me, it's the magic on the journey. Too many people get obsessed with the 'end point', thinking that the happiness comes upon achieving the goal. Whilst that is true to some extent, never underestimate the great things that happen along the way.

Back in 2019, with my boys sleeping through the night and my health and fitness fully underway, I set a big goal. I wanted to run the Cardiff half-marathon aged forty-one. My goal was to reach the finish line in under 1 hour 38 mins, hopefully dropping some unwanted weight along the way.

Don't ask me why I picked that time, but I just knew that if I did it, it would have to be at least ten minutes quicker than anything I'd done before.

Remember I told you about how deflated I'd become when I dropped out of races when my boys were young? Remember the 'banter' I'd gotten from the boot camp lads for always dropping out of races? I promised myself I would make the comeback stronger and this goal time was perfect for me.

I wrote the goal down and reflected on it. I thought back to those early days of fatherhood; how I truly believed my best days were behind me.

I then recalled the time when I could run those half marathons with ease. I would fly across that finish line with a massive smile on my face.

I had run many Cardiff half-marathons before. I knew the course inside out and I knew the exact route to the finish line.

I planted a vision in my head of me breezing home at forty-one, lean and fit again after some very tough years. I also wrote out the following on a piece of paper and carried it around with me in my wallet:

"On Saturday 5th October 2019 I will weigh 85kgs. This will equate to a loss of around 6kgs. This will be the lightest and leanest I have been since my first son John came along seven years ago."

"On Sunday 6th October 2019, I will run the quickest time I have ever done in a half marathon event at Cardiff. My goal is sub 1 hour 38 minutes."

"When I achieve this goal, it will feel amazing

because I have proved to myself I can still get lean at almost forty-one years of age. I will also prove to myself that I can run the fastest half marathon I have ever done since becoming a dad seven years ago."

This visualisation fired me up. It kept me focused and made me do the work. Even on days when motivation was low, I still monitored my calories, trained and stayed off the booze.

The day before the race, I weighed in at 11lbs lighter.

Why?

Well, the big goal had kept me focused. It helped me to consistently keep doing the work. Doing the work consistently led to weight loss.

Another huge driving factor was knowing that if I could get lighter and leaner before the race, it would help me to run quicker.

All these factors combined, led to me feeling the best I had in years. And that was even before the race, when I just lining up at the start line!

I ran the race, felt great and came home in just over 1hr and 38 minutes, missing my target by about 45 seconds.

Was I disappointed? Hell no!

I'd set a big goal that I'd gotten nowhere near

for the past seven years; a goal that scared the life out of me!

I also told everyone in advance what I was trying to achieve. That put some pressure on me and made me super accountable. I cannot stress how important these factors were to making me do the work.

When I crossed the finish line that day, the sense of achievement was incredible. It had been a long road back after years of sleepless nights and hospital visits with the boys. This meant much more to me than just crossing the line in a decent time.

I was also proving to myself that I could do it at 40+ let alone 30+.

I'd gained two stone after the kids were born. There were times I felt like a fraud; how could I build this dream fitness business when I felt overweight? There were times I was so exhausted, that I questioned myself. Would I ever be able to come back strong?

Finishing the Cardiff half-marathon in 2019, weighing in at a decent 85kgs and feeling lean again, was the catalyst to start writing this book. I had finally regained confidence and believed I had something to offer.

If you think you can rely on motivation to achieve your goal, then think again.

Motivation will get you started, but when it runs out (and it will), you'll need a clear goal that really means something to you.

I say this to all new clients: Can you consider doing some sort of physical challenge which will stimulate you, scare you a little and get you out of your comfort zone?

It could be a half marathon.

It could be a hill walk.

It could be a long-distance bike ride.

Don't do something that doesn't light a fire in you, because when the going gets tough, you simply won't see it through. Cardiff half-marathon 2019 meant so much to me for all the reasons I have mentioned above.

Could the commitment needed for your challenge encourage and force you to make positive lifestyle changes? Changes that, in turn, will lead to weight loss?

The by-product of committing to such an event is that you improve health, fitness and get leaner. Once you are clear on what it is, then go ahead and sign up!

The next step is: Tell everybody! Honestly,

this has always worked for me because it adds another layer of accountability.

I always announce what challenges I'm doing on social media, because I know that for every ten people that want me to succeed, there will be one that wants me to fail. I fucking love that.

Knowing that someone out there wants me to fail is a massive driver for me. Psychologically, it always works when the tough gets going.

Finally, for that ultra-level of accountability, I will pick a charity to run for.

A charity that I have done a lot of events for over the years is the Noah's Ark Children's Hospital for Wales. They looked after my boys on multiple occasions throughout their early years.

The thought of not wanting to let them down after I had raised money, combined with the thought of proving the doubters wrong, has spurred me on, both in training and during the event itself. Of course, there is the added driver of wanting to make my loved ones proud.

I read a fantastic quote a few years back and it said: "It's easy to fail in private, it's not easy to fail in public." This is why I just love to tell the world my goals. I encourage you guys to do the same!

If goals are a great motivator, then what is even greater?

Habits and systems

Habits and systems: something I never considered much until I read a book called "Atomic Habits" by author James Clear.

Habits and systems are the two things which are absolutely key in transforming your life (and body) for the better.

When I first read this book, it completely threw me. I had always preached about setting big goals, writing them down and visualizing them. Then James Clear came along and said: "Whilst goals help us win a game, it's habits and systems that keep us playing the game."

He went on to say that most humans have a distorted view of their own behaviour, meaning – we think we behave better than we do. We believe we eat less than we actually do. We think we drink less alcohol than we tell others.

Taking exact measurements, is therefore one way to overcome our blindness.

This made so much sense to me. I thought about my clients and how alarmed they would become when they realise how much they actually eat. When they download My Fitness Pal and start to track calories, it comes as a major shock.

In the same vein, they also become alarmed when they purchase a fitness tracker and see how little they move! They put it on their wrist and are shocked to discover they're doing much less than their expected 3,000 steps a day.

I often say: "What gets measured, gets managed." This saying was coined after reading Clear's book.

Why are habits and systems so important? Why is it simply not enough to have a big goal?

Well, as James Clear says, everyone has goals, but not everyone achieves them.

Let's take, for example, two football teams in a cup final. Both teams, having come so far, will have the goal of winning on the day, but only one team will end up winning.

What's the difference? Luck can play a part, but it will also boil down to preparation, tactics and a plan (ie: systems).

The team that wins the cup, not only had the goal of winning the cup, but had the systems and habits in place to earn that success.

This may seem hard to grasp. It can feel as

though habits and systems make very little impact on any given day. However, over time, the impact is enormous.

Think about it.

Most of us will have, at some point, joined a gym. We will have followed a plan and expected results in two weeks. When the results did not come immediately, it was easy to let it slide or sack it off completely.

On the other hand, if we had just followed it for 4-6 months, the results may have been life changing and set us off on a whole new trajectory.

"Be concerned about your current trajectory and not your current results," James added.

You see, the slow pace of transformation makes habits easy to slide. It's human nature to give up when instant change is not seen.

James went on to add: "The goal is not to just run the race; the goal is to become the runner. Long after the race is over, you continue to follow the habits and systems that the runner would."

Therefore, when it comes to fat loss, the goal shouldn't be to get to your desired outcome as quickly as possible. It should be about enjoying the process.

The goal should be: Become the person who not only loses the weight, but does it in a way that's easy to maintain. It can then be continually maintained, long after the goal is achieved.

Let me give you an example:–

I am currently 83kgs.

Let's say my goal is to get to 79kgs.

I could probably do this in around two weeks like this:–

- Aggressive calorie deficit (upwards of 1250 cal deficit a day)
- Extremely low carbs
- No alcohol or junk food
- Lots of cardio
- 20k steps a day
- 5 litres water a day

The results? I'd be miserable, irritable and lacking in energy. I wouldn't enjoy the experience; I'd merely be waiting to hit the magical 79kg on the scale.

Then, the moment I hit my goal; I would probably rebound aggressively.

However, if I continue to follow my current habits and systems, it might take me two months rather than two weeks, but the process would be much more enjoyable.

- Manageable 250-500 deficit a day
- Plenty of carbs
- Alcohol and a takeaway on the weekend (factored in)
- Normal workouts with gym, kettle bells and 7-aside (no need for extra cardio)
- 15k steps a day
- 2-3 litres water a day

The above is what I do day-to-day with enjoyment and ease.

Carrying on this way with consistency, will take me to my goal and then keep me maintaining, simply because the daily habits and systems remain the same.

Remember that achieving a goal is only a momentary change. It changes your life for the moment only. Therefore, we need to enjoy the journey because this is what we will be on the most.

To conclude I want you to ask yourself:–

- What is my goal and why is it so important to me?

Saying "I want to lose 20lbs" is not enough. You don't just want lose 20lb, you want the <u>feeling</u> that comes with losing 20 pounds –:

- Increased energy
- Increased self-confidence
- Feeling better in clothes

Now sit and visualise for a second:–

- Why is this important to me?
- How will I feel when I achieve this goal?
- What will my friends and family think when I achieve this goal?
- How will achieving this goal benefit my life?
- How will I walk, talk and behave when I achieve this goal?

I want you to ask yourself these questions and answer them in as much detail as you can.

- What do I need to do in order to achieve my goal sensibly whilst enjoying the journey?
- How long will this take?
- What new daily habits do I need to make in order to achieve this goal?

- What do I need to give up or reduce in order to achieve my goal?
- How prepared am I to give up or reduce those things in order to achieve my goal?
- What is more important?
- What habits or behaviors do I need to reduce or give up in order to achieve my goal?
- Why is my goal more important than the habits (or behaviors) I need to reduce or give up?
- Can I achieve my goal using the new daily habits when motivation ultimately runs out?

Write down your goal, create the systems and habits, tell people, get accountable and give yourself time.

Motivation will run dry, but a clear goal + habits and systems will keep you in play.

CHAPTER FOURTEEN

Fat loss pills – anxiety and depression

As WE GET TOWARDS the latter end of this book, I feel it's only fair to tell you about my experience of using fat burners, which in turn, led to anxiety and depression.

I'm sure I can give you enough information to warn you away from this dangerous road. Trust me when I say I would not want anyone to experience what I went through. It is, however, part of my journey, and hence why I have included it.

From the age of nine or ten upwards, my weight was always up and down. I look back at old photos and see that my weight was never constant. Sure, I had periods where I was trim and happy. Between the ages of twelve to seventeen was when I was the most consistent.

I discovered cross-country running at secondary school and it was the first time I had really stood out at anything. I joined the local athletic club in Gloucester where I began to excel at 1500 meters and cross-country. It was an amazing time in my life. I was well-liked and supported. I also got to train with a great bunch of runners, several times a week.

I soon became district champion and country runner-up. As a result of all the training I was doing, I was extremely trim. It had a knock-on effect on my football too. As my endurance continued to build, I felt that my game picked up.

Most weekends I would have a race on a Saturday, followed by footy on a Sunday. I loved it. These were happy times and I have very fond memories.

Then, around the age of sixteen or seventeen, like most of us, I discovered alcohol. Dropping off the competitive running, I started to enjoy weekend drinks with my mates. Needless to say, I started to gain some weight.

It was when I moved to university in Wales, that I gained loads of weight for the first time in years. Student life; drinking five nights a week and enjoying regular takeaways, really took its toll.

By the second year, I had discovered Cardiff night life, a local lady and some party chemicals. I was soon dancing my way to visible abs. The summer of 1999 (which I call the summer of love), I was at my leanest ever, simply from cutting shapes at Cardiff's dance clubs.

However, my weight never stayed the same; it was always up or down. From the ages of twenty to twenty-six, my weight fluctuated massively.

I was a nightclub and event promoter at the time; working long weekends, drinking loads and eating late night burgers. Don't get me wrong, I was always active. I would either go out running, play 5-a-side, or mess around in the gym. However, I was clueless as to what I should be doing.

Weight was a constant battle and at that stage, I wasn't ready to accept the extent of my poor relationship with food.

Around the age of twenty-seven however, I was to discover something: *Ephedrine*. Once I took it, it made me feel invincible. I felt like it would finally rid me of my weight problems.

I was due to go to Cuba with my partner at the time for a two-week all-inclusive. We had gone on many of these over the years, and like I said, my weight was either up or down. When I went to the Cayman Islands back in 2002, it was a real low point for me, weight-wise. I felt really fat.

By the time we visited the Dominican Republic a year later, I had lost almost three stone by playing a LOT of 5-a-side.

After that, there were a few years of the weight going up and down. I never cracked it and it was an on-going battle.

Five weeks before I was due to travel to Cuba, I started to panic. I needed to lose weight, and fast! A friend told me about ephedrine and got some for me. However, he warned that they were pretty hard-core.

If you've never heard of ephedrine, it's now a banned substance. Diego Maradona was banned from the World Cup in 1994 for taking it.

I took my first one before a run. It blew my fucking head off!

Within thirty minutes, I was shaking and tingling. I ended up completing an awesome run. Despite being heavy, I was able to run hard. The sweat was pouring out of me.

I was also wearing a bin liner underneath my clothes because I heard it made you sweat more. Boy, it did!

I took an ephedrine, ripped a few holes in a

bin liner to get my head and arms in, tucked it into my shorts, put a top on, and off I went.

When I got back from the run, I took my shirt off and ripped open the biner liner. A large puddle of sweat poured out.

I genuinely thought this was doing me good, when in fact, all I was doing was losing water.

I was still clueless about nutrition, but ephedrine curbed my appetite, so in my eyes, it was a double-win!

There were days I would wake, feeling like I was on a comedown from party chemicals. However, I'd simply pop another ephedrine and within thirty minutes, I'd feel lively enough for another run. (I cringe as I remember this!)

I was running five days of the week and not eating much. At the time, I didn't know it, but I was creating a massive calorie deficit. I lost a lot of weight. I must have dropped between 14-20lbs in a five-week period before that holiday.

With taking ephedrine, I'd gotten used to the jitters. I also developed horrendous road rage. At the time, I was driving a van and working as a courier. My head would blow in traffic! Along with that, was the dry mouth. And to top it all off, I had a stinging sensation every time I would pee.

But hey ho, I was losing weight, right?

I got to Cuba, hit the beach, and actually felt half decent about myself.

Looking back at photos, I can see that I had gotten pretty trim, however I was by no means "lean". I had certainly dropped a lot of fat (as well as muscle).

On that holiday, I ate and drank to my heart's content. I was loving life. In two weeks, I gained half a stone. But hey, with all-inclusive, it's easily done, right?

However, upon returning from the holiday, the weight still kept creeping on.

I was out of ephedrine. As my body fat started to increase, so did my desire to pop the ephedrine.

It was when I started taking them again, that I suffered my first ever panic attack.

I had grown accustomed to the side effects to some degree. However, I couldn't bear how irritable I was when driving my work van. If I got stuck in traffic, my patience was non-existent. My head would blow.

After a busy day in the van, the traffic was unbearable. I could feel myself getting wound up. However, this time it was worse – I started to get really bad hot flushes.

I hadn't experienced anything like it before and it made me feel breathless and panicky. The flushes were travelling up the back of my neck and tingling around my head. Nervous, I started to think it was the ephedrine.

My mates had always warned me: "It'll come back to bite you on the arse!"

Of course, when you're losing weight and having loads of energy, you don't care! I went home that night, crashed out on the sofa and told myself that after a good night's sleep, I'd be fine.

The next day, I still had the hot flushes.

Driving around in the van for work, I started to feel very, very anxious.

I had rolled all the windows down to get fresh air, but the feeling was getting more and more intense.

I hadn't told my partner at the time about the ephedrine, but I remember telling myself I would never going near them again.

The panicky feeling carried on for several days and by then, I was really starting to worry. It was completely overwhelming.

I was driving around in my van, totally consumed with fear and it was only getting worse.

I was on a pick-up at around 4pm at a place called SA Brains. The hot flushes were beyond manageable and the feeling of panic was rising. I genuinely started to think I was having a heart attack.

Scared shitless and tearful, I said to the lady on reception: "Can you please get me a medic? I'm feeling really sick. I think I'm about to have a heart attack!"

It was horrific.

A young medic (who had probably done only a few hours of training in her life), led me to a chair and sat with me. As I sat down, I could feel my legs starting to go numb. Then a feeling of pins and needles travelled up from my feet.

By this stage, I had moved onto the floor, lying in terror while people in the office crowded around, calling an ambulance and relaying questions back and forth.

"Any heart conditions in the family?"

"Are on you any medication?"

"How old are you?"

I lay there, firmly believing my time was up.

Twenty-six years old, lying there in horror, thinking: "I'm done, I'm dead."

The pins and needles continued to travel up

my body and had reached my stomach and chest. Three quarters of my body was locked up, unable to move.

I was thinking: *'Any minute now. This is the moment I'm going to die.'*

I was waiting for it to take me out.

Next thing, a couple of paramedics turned up. They took one look at me on the floor and said: "Hey bud. It's alright, mate."

They grabbed me by the hand, very matter of fact, and said: "Come on up! You're not having a heart attack. You've got a lot of colour in your face. If you were having a heart attack, you'd be grey."

"It's not a heart attack you're having – it's a panic attack."

They then tried to walk with me around the car park!

The funny thing is, my whole body was locked up. As they tried to walk me around the car park, I was like a robot – like fucking C3P0 out of Star Wars. I could barely move!

However, as they continued to get me to walk slowly, the blood flow must've returned to my legs and I began to loosen up.

In my frightened and overwhelmed state, I

admitted: "I've been taking ephedrine!"

The paramedic paused, looked at me and, very matter of fact, said: "Well, that's not going to help, is it?"

They put the blue lights on and whizzed me off to hospital for checks. Thankfully, everything was fine. The nurses had been informed that I'd been taking extreme weight loss supplements. They gave me a little pep talk (deservedly), warning me not to take them again.

I checked out of hospital that night feeling shaky, disorientated and relieved.

My partner and family knew I'd had a panic attack, but they probably didn't know the extent of my ephedrine consumption.

"I'm never ever doing that again," I told myself. To this day, I've never touched them.

Whilst I'd like to tell you that this was the end of saga, it was only just the beginning.

The next day I woke up, still jittery and anxious. Whilst I was relieved I hadn't had a heart attack, I couldn't ignore these feelings. In the following months, I developed a sensation of feeling off-balance, almost as if I was on a ship. It was awful and made my anxiety worse.

I was back at work and driving around in my

van. I had to keep a brown paper bag handy in case another panic attack came on.

I can't explain just how awful it was to have this feeling of being off balance and slightly dizzy all the time. It started to take over my life, affect my sleep and my relationship. I was a nervous wreck and often bursting into tears.

I was convinced I'd done some major damage to myself and started to seek help. Using my private health insurance, I booked in to see an Ear, Nose and throat specialist, as well as a neurologist.

They couldn't find anything wrong with me, so the next port of call was a cardiologist for a C.T. scan. I was convinced I may have damaged my heart with long-term ephedrine use, but it came back all-clear.

In fact, upon scanning me, the cardiologist said that he would 'happily swap hearts' with me. One positive!

Despite getting the all-clear from all these experts, the feelings of being off-balance persisted. I was in a very dark place, full of anxiety and worry.

I came across a website that offered support for people with dizziness. It only made matters worse because everyone ended up diagnosing each other!

One day, I could see no way out. I was in floods of tears and didn't want to live like this anymore. The anxiety was way too much.

I put a cry for help in the group and the support I received was incredible. Someone in the group recommended a top 'balance' specialist. He was living in South Wales and I managed to get an appointment with him. I was delighted to be meeting an expert in the field.

I laid my soul bear to him, telling him how lost and confused I felt. I confessed that I was worried I'd make matters worse by attempting exercise. I was concerned about my future and felt like I was running out of places to turn.

He listened closely and went on to explain that I was suffering from something called 'Peripheral vestibular dysfunction'. It was an imbalance between my ears that could have been brought on by using ephedrine.

He went on to explain that my anxiety about the situation would only heighten the symptoms and make me feel worse.

Whenever I'd been exercising, I was thinking: *'I'm gonna die. I'm gonna keel over any minute.'* This was not only consuming me, but making it ten times worse.

He then set me free by saying: "Continue to play sports and exercise. Whatever makes you dizzy, makes you better."

This was a massive sense of relief to me as I'd been living off my nerves for months.

I went away on a high and tried to get on with life, even though the symptoms prevailed.

The consultant's words rang in my ears: 'The symptoms will take time to disappear until one day you'll realize they're less severe or they have just passed.'

I tried to carry on with things. Looking back, the symptoms did start to ease, but then things took another turn for the worse.

I had a pretty heavy weekend on the beers with some friends and was feeling pretty rough on the Sunday. I told myself I'd be fine after a good night's sleep. However, when I woke on Monday, despite having a really long night's sleep, I felt completely exhausted. It was almost as if I hadn't slept at all. Not only did I feel exhausted, but I felt really tearful.

I tried to go about my day even though I felt absolutely knackered. I told myself that if I got another good night's sleep, I'd be okay. I wasn't.

I got another solid night's sleep and again, woke up feeling like I hadn't. Instead of nerve-racking anxiety, I was drained and in floods of tears.

I had slipped into (what I now know was) depression.

I firmly believe that a number of things had caught up with me: years of battling my weight, yo-yo dieting, using ephedrine and other party chemicals. I think there were a few other factors at play too, but I'd like to keep them private.

I went to see my doctor and broke down. I'd been no stranger to seeing her over the years and she'd been a really good source of support.

She said: "Mark, I've seen you on-and-off for a few years. You live on your nerves. I think you need something to make you more stable."

She recommended an anti-depressant called Citalopram and said it would help me feel more level. I was very, very nervous about taking it, but I did take it.

I started off with twenty milligrams, and then at one stage moved up to forty.

I felt very sick when I started on them. I had been told to give it a few weeks before I noticed any changes. However, hand on heart, I started to feel the difference within seven to ten days.

Now, I'm not a doctor. I wouldn't recommend anyone else to take them, but all I'll say is, they helped me a lot. What also helped me, was that I had a very loving, supportive partner at the time.

Once the medication kicked in, I felt the emotional exhaustion and crippling anxiety had lifted. I was finally able to move on with my life.

There had been times during that awful period where I didn't even want to leave the house. I had been in such a bad place, but thankfully I had a loving partner. She used to always encourage me to go out for walks with her, and sure enough, I'd always feel better afterwards.

Looking back now at my twenty-six-year-old self, I don't even recognize that guy. However, in a way, I'm glad I had that experience because it made me who I am today.

I know how it feels to be anxious, I know how it feels to be depressed, and I know how crippling it is to wake up exhausted and emotional. That was, hands down, the worst time of my life, but it made me.

I believe it's the reason why I have a deeper empathy with my clients. I have been there, got the tee shirt and know how it feels to be suicidal.

The antidepressants kicked in and the ephedrine never touched my lips again. It wasn't long before my eureka moment – my decision to enter the fitness industry. A decision which was to change my life forever.

It was time to fix myself properly and then be able to help others.

CHAPTER FIFTEEN

The Law of Attraction

YOU MIGHT BE THINKING: *What the hell is it and why is it in this book?*

If you have come this far and are enjoying the information I'm giving you, then I hope you trust me enough to listen to what I'm about to tell you. Just roll with it!

I could not write this book without including my journey into the world of self-development and spirituality.

Before I teach my clients any of this stuff, I ask them to simply keep an open mind! If I have helped to open your eyes to health and fitness, then let me put the icing on the cake!

By now, you already know about my weight battles in the past; my experience with fat burners, panic attacks, anxiety and depression. These all played a part in my life up until the age of twenty-six or twenty-seven.

It's fair to say that I was all over the place and not a happy soul. At times, I thought the world owed me a favour. I was snappy, anxious and easily wound up. No doubt the ephedrine was the main contributor, however I really believed that bad luck followed me around.

During my time working as a self-employed courier, my van was always having problems. It seemed like I was always shelling out to have it repaired. I was constantly forking out cash on a van that continued to let me down.

Not only was I angry with the van, I was angry I didn't know what to do with my life! Well-meaning but hurtful comments from friends really pissed me off. They always said I should be doing something better with my life.

For some reason, I just expected bad luck. I assumed that things wouldn't go my way.

Mum, who had been very worried about me, handing me a book called 'The Secret' by an Australian author called Rhonda Byrne. It was late 2005, a short time before I had my life-changing moment. To say that this book changed my life completely would be an understatement, however it didn't happen straight away.

The book came with accompanying CD's.

Mum suggested I should listen to them whilst driving along in the van. After all, I had used the long-distance driving time to learn Spanish, why didn't I listen to this and see where it took me?

Mum told me that all I had to do, was keep an open mind.

You can imagine the scene. I was about twenty-five years old and not in a good place. I was overweight and anxious. My van kept breaking down and I didn't have any direction in life.

Driving along, I put the CD on for the first time. The introduction was all this spiritual, chiming music. Then a voice started to whisper: "I want to tell you a secret."

I was like; "For fuck's sake! What is this bollocks?" I snapped it off straightaway.

It really wound me up and I told my mum: "It's not for me."

Life continued as it was for a few weeks; the same hum-drum drudgery. The thought occurred to me that maybe I should contemplate trying out that CD again.

I thought: "Well, what have I got to lose?"

Afterall, I was driving around in the van, anxious and uptight. Life wasn't how I wanted it to be. What harm would it do to give the thing a listen? I was looking for something, anything to give me some direction.

After we got over the spiritual music and the weird whispering, it started to talk about this fascinating subject of the Law of Attraction.

Basically; what we think about, we attract.

The narrator explained that most of us attract things we don't want because it's all we think about.

- Money problems
- Relationship problems
- Work problems

The list goes on.

It started to make me think about how negative my mindset was. If this law was true, then I was responsible for all the shit that was going wrong in my life.

The narrator then went on to talk about gratitude.

Remember how I said I was always going around angry and upset, thinking the world owed me a favour? When I listen about the power of gratitude, I realized I was never grateful.

The audio explained that if you change your mindset from self-pity to gratitude, then your world begins to change.

It explained that no matter how bad we think our life is, we always have something to be grateful for. I liked this because it wasn't too spiritual for me; it just sounded like common sense. It unlocked a different way of thinking for the first time ever.

I thought: 'Okay, I may hate my job, but I'm grateful for a caring partner who puts up with me. I'm grateful I've got money coming in. I'm grateful for my family who care about me.'

A really warm and fuzzy feeling came over me. I simply hadn't taken the time to devise a list like this before. I can do this!

The book encouraged to start each day by being grateful for a few things. You could write them down, say them aloud, or simply think them.

What happens when you get past the big stuff, like being grateful for family, a roof over your head and a loving partner? You could simply list three smaller things.

It could be that you were grateful for a good night sleep, a warm bed to wake up in and a morning coffee.

I liked this concept – I really liked it. I also had

nothing to lose. So, I started to be grateful.

It simply started to put me in a better mood each morning!

I was now focused on what I DID have, rather than on what I didn't. As I drove along in my van, I listened to the CD over and over on a daily basis. It encouraged me not to feel angry at things that happen, but rather, to be grateful. It was about re-framing everything. Rather than being pissed off about paying a bill, it suggested I try to be grateful for the service I was provided.

This was tricky at first, but I was willing to give it a go. I was convinced that gratitude was genuinely making me happier.

The next time I had to shell out for my van and buy a new tyre, I tried to re-frame my thinking. Instead of being pissed off at the cost, I would feel grateful that my van was road-safe.

Things started to gently change in my life. It was shortly after this, that I had my eureka moment whilst running the 10k race in Bute Park, Cardiff.

Was this down to me changing my thought processes? Was this down to me being more grateful? Or was this simply down to a conversation with my friend Ralph who was thinking of becoming a personal trainer – a conversation that planted a seed?

Either way, it wasn't long after dabbling with a new way of thinking, that my life was about to change completely.

I don't want you to think it was complete plain sailing from then on, because it wasn't. Despite practicing gratitude, the anxiety still plagued me. I still didn't believe in myself. It took me to push past the fear during that first weekend on the course, to break free from the anxiety that consumed me.

Once I got past that weekend and realized that everyone on my course were normal folk just like me, I was able to keep going. After that, I started to delve deeper into the teaching of the Secret and the Law of Attraction.

I started to learn about the subject of visualisation. This was the next stage on from practicing gratitude. Visualisation is a method whereby you imagine vividly how you want your life to become.

Like I said, most people are going around thinking about what they DON'T want, rather than what they DO want.

Visualisation is tough. It can be hard to even

dare to dream of how you want your life to turn out. After all, most of us are complete sceptics!

I was finding it hard to visualise until I got past that first weekend of the course. Then an interesting thing happened.

I was still working as a courier and up to my eyes studying to become a personal trainer. I was also slowly getting into the Law of Attraction. I had to go to a local warehouse to pick up a parcel. When I arrived, there was a guy in front of me in the queue, also waiting for a package.

He was about ten years older than me, wearing a tracksuit and in awesome shape. I presumed he must work in fitness. I nervously struck up a conversation with him. It turned out he was a personal trainer and was there to pick up some resistance bands.

I told him that I was training to be a personal trainer. He wasn't overly friendly or chatty. However, I watched as he left the premises, jumped into a beautiful sports car and drove off. That was the visual I needed.

There he was, in great shape, wearing a designer tracksuit and driving a lovely sports car.

I said to myself there and then, "I'm going to be that guy."

As I studied to become a personal trainer, I held onto that vision, day-in and day-out.

Fast forward two years, I had a moment of clarity. I was a full-time personal trainer, owned a growing business and had lost weight. Remember how I told you about my mate Lee who was a car salesman? He insisted I needed a nice sports car to reflect the fruits of my labour. He suggested the Audi TT and sorted the finance for me.

I realized I was now that guy! In a career I loved, in control of my weight and driving a sports car! A few years before, it was a scenario I would never have dreamt possible.

I had become what I had visualized. It hit me all of sudden; so much so that I became over-whelmed with emotion and gratitude.

I was totally convinced by this Law of Attraction stuff, but I was only scratching the surface. Now that I was living with my friend Lee and out of a long-term relationship, I started to delve deeper and became more aware of what could be possible.

In the space of two years, I'd gone from being lost and hating life, to super focused and loving life. I was also earning a few quid, something I hadn't even considered when entering the industry.

I got busy very quickly and was often coaching seven days a week. Moving forward, I knew I needed to work smarter if I was ever going to have a family.

After listening to some gurus in the States (and following them online), I had the inspired idea of setting up an over 30's Boot camp for men. '30-plus fitness' was born.

The Boot camp kicked off and it was great fun. It enabled me to train more people at once, charge less and work less hours. It also gave me a bit more work/life balance, which is what I had been looking for.

Learning about the Law of Attraction had served me well, so I started to read about the 'Secret to wealth' – how to attract money.

Money was never my primary intention when contemplating a career change. However, not only was I doing something I loved, I was also earning about £30k a year from one-to-one coaching. This was a figure I would only have dreamt about in the past.

The teaching of the Secret kept saying;

- Set a financial goal that both scares and excites you
- Write it down

- Provide value in your services every day
- Let the universe do the rest.

It was the gurus in the States that I had been listening to, who inspired me to set up my boot camps. They kept saying that you could earn six figures a year running boot camps. I was like: "Six Figures? That's like £100k a year! That's simply not possible!"

However, despite my skepticism, I was already convinced it worked. After all, miracles were already happening in my own life.

This was simply going to require a higher level of thinking, visualising and believing.

I sat down and worked out the Maths. £100k per year would equate to £8,333 per month. I would need around eighty Boot campers a month to get to that magical number.

I'd never even considered it before, but it planted a seed.

I only had about ten members in my boot camp at the time. Eighty seemed so unattainable, but I decided to have some fun with it.

The Secret recommended writing down your goals and repeating them as affirmations every morning. So, I sat down with a piece of paper and wrote an affirmation:

"I'm so happy and grateful right now, that I love what I do and I have created a six-figure boot camp by (date*). Thank you, thank you, thank you."

(* I think I gave myself about a year.)

It felt crazy, but I pinned it up on my bedroom wall. Every morning when I woke up, I would look at it. I'd repeat the affirmation, whilst feeling grateful for the life I was currently enjoying.

It was easy because I was genuinely very grateful for the life I had at that present moment in time.

I would repeat it again whilst I was driving along in my car. When I went out running, I would repeat it again. Sometimes I'd say it out loud, sometimes I would just think it in my head, but I always felt good when I said it.

It wasn't even about the money. I didn't need six figures to be happy. I'd found happiness in my career. I was just curious to see if this could work on a bigger level.

I continued to show up every day and add value to my clients' lives. Meanwhile, I continued to feel grateful, visualised and repeated the same affirmation.

My 30+ Boot camp was launched in May 2010.

By Christmas that year, I had hit around twenty-five members which I was extremely happy with. However, it was nowhere near the eighty I needed if I wanted to reach that six-figure income.

Occasionally, my 30+ lads would ask me if I did a boot camp for ladies. I would just say no. I was honestly happy with my PT business and a growing 30+ boot camp. There was an amazing atmosphere in our solid and exciting niche.

However, by Christmas 2010, I was being asked several times a week. Boot camp for ladies? Boot camp for ladies?

As Christmas was fast approaching and people were thinking about their new year's resolutions, I suppose a lot of the lads had partners who wanted to get fit too.

The lads were practically begging me to run classes for the ladies and offering to pay for their partner. I simply couldn't keep saying no. With so many men asking for help with fitness for their other halves, it would have been ridiculous to turn it down.

So, I was like: "Okay! I'll do something!"

I put a post on Facebook the day after boxing day. I worded it in a similar manner as I had done with the 30+ ad. I said that I was looking for ten ladies who wanted to be part of a female only (non-intimidating) boot-camp in the new year.

The response was phenomenal. On the first Wednesday night of January 2011, thirty-seven girls turned up. 'Booty camp' was born.

We didn't even have a name at the time. The girls named it themselves later on in the month. By the end of that month, I had about forty members.

By February 2011, between my two boot camps, I now had eighty members.

Combined with my personal training business, I had reached the £8,333 per month = equating to a £100k per year income.

My mind was blown. Realising how much this stuff had worked, I cried tears of joy.

For years I had suffered with anxiety and depression. It was only four years before that I had that eureka moment and decided to face my fears and enter the fitness industry.

I was now thirty-two years old with a six-figure business; something I would never have even fathomed possible. Becoming awakened to what was possible had dramatically changed my life.

None of this is to impress you.

If you have come this far, you will know about my biggest struggles. You will also know about my values in life. Money was never a key driver for me; I simply wanted to be happy. I'd simply wanted a career I could be passionate about.

A business coach once said to me: "Tregs, don't chase money. Just show up every day and add value. Be passionate and the money will chase you."

He was so right.

Remember I told you I had written down: *I am so grateful to have a six-figure boot camp business?*

I never stated that it'd be solely from "30+" men. I merely stated that it would be "Boot camp." The universe provided the opportunity to set up a Ladies boot camp and it happened within a few short months (not a year!). The six-figure boot camp had been manifested.

It blew my mind.

By this stage, I was completely convinced that the Law of Attraction worked. I was ready to delve even deeper. I couldn't believe how much my life had changed and how happy I was. The more I practiced gratitude and more I visualised, the better life became!

After a short-term relationship with a girl from overseas that didn't work out, I settled into my own apartment in Cardiff Bay. I was loving life. I had affirmations everywhere; on the fridge, on the bathroom mirror, in my wallet. There were reminders all over the place of how I wanted my life to become.

The joy of living on my own was that there was no resistance to any of it. I didn't worry that a partner would think I was crazy. Most days, I was bellowing affirmations out loud. It felt fucking amazing.

So, life was going well and business was growing. I had a lovely apartment in Cardiff Bay and a nice sports car. However, I'd been single for about a year and I was starting to think it would be nice to meet someone.

"The Secret" doesn't only cover career and money, there's also an entire chapter devoted to relationships. Because I could see how it had worked for every other aspect of my life, I was all ears.

The book spoke about creating room in your life for someone, if that is what you wanted. You might say that you want a relationship, but have you created the space in your life for one? Is there

space for someone else's clothes in your wardrobe? Would they have a parking space?

It all sounds a bit crazy, right?

However, because I could see how much this
stuff worked for my business and career, I had
faith it would work for relationships too.

I had been dating a few women and enjoying
myself, however I hadn't met anyone that I totally
clicked with.

I listened to the audio which asked if I had
made room in my home for someone. Suddenly,
it hit me in the face! I still had my ex-partner's
dressing gown and a few of her dresses hanging
in my wardrobe!

I rushed home, packed up my ex-partner's
clothes and flung them into a charity shop the
following day.

Just a few days later, I was chatting to a couple of ladies on the dating website: Match.com. A
friend had randomly recommended it to me a few
weeks previously.

I got chatting to a girl called Sarah. She told
me she had noticed my profile, but hadn't
messaged. Her reason? My profile stated that my
age preference was someone younger than
myself. At the time, I was thirty-two and she was
thirty-seven!

We carried on chatting and she said: "I'm sure I know your face. Do you go to the 'Train Station 2' gym?"

It turned out that she was living only one mile away from me. She went to the same gym I coached at and her personal trainer was one of my friends! She joked that in the gym, she was always able to hear me before she saw me! The more we chatted, we talked about going out for a drink.

There was only one thing that didn't sit right with me.

There's an unwritten rule that you don't get romantically involved with friend's clients in the industry. I wanted to talk to Jason first to check he was okay with it. When I caught up with him, I told him that I'd been chatting to one of his clients on an online dating site. When I mentioned Sarah's name, he was totally cool with it. He even remarked that she was a great laugh and we would hit it off.

We arranged a date at Starbucks in the Bay.

I turned up in my black Audi TT, thinking I was the absolute nuts, dressed like something out of a fucking boy band!

She turned up a bit late and got out of a silver

BMW. I was like; *"Ooooft! I'm in trouble here!"*

She looked absolutely stunning. I remember thinking, "I'm way out of my league. I'm gonna need to depend on my personality to pull this one off!"

We had a great laugh and got on fantastically. To cut a very long story short, we were practically living together after a couple of weeks. Within a few months, I had given up my apartment to officially move in with her.

We met in April 2011, moved in together by August 2011, and by November 2011, she was pregnant with our first baby, John. We were over the moon.

Considering we were both in our thirties, we'd had the 'kids' chat very early on in our relationship. With Sarah being five years older than me, we didn't want to waste our time!

Ten years on and with two beautiful kids, I still marvel at the circumstances that brought us together. Was it the Law of Attraction? Whole-heartedly, I believe YES, it was!

I firmly believe that practicing the techniques in that book allowed her to walk into my life. It also opened the door for two beautiful boys, who bring me more joy than I could have ever wished for.

I have used the Law of Attraction multiple times over the years to manifest miracles into my life. Anything from; unexpected income, to new clients, to going global online, to amazing podcast guests. It never fails me!

However, I will say, that you have to immerse yourself in it, every day. You have to do the work – and it isn't always easy! As you know, we had two kids very quickly. Life changed practically overnight for me. There was a lot of pressure on my shoulders in a very short space of time. This, coupled with constant tiredness in the kids' early years, meant that I stopped practicing the Law of Attraction for a few years.

You see, it's very easy to do when you feel good, but not so easy to do so when you feel tired!

However, once the kids started to sleep the whole night through, I decided to make a physical comeback. I also decided to make a mental comeback and began practicing the Law of Attraction again.

One of the things I always do now is: **Give.**

I love giving to charity. Giving is one of the greatest things you can do, to show the universe that you are ready to receive. It shows that you have an abundant mindset and don't fear lack.

Guess what? Every time I give, good things happen to me. Not necessarily from the person I gave to – it doesn't work like that. However, the universe always finds a way of delivering it back via someone or something.

It's a lesson I try to pass on my kids. If you can help others less fortunate than you and do it without expectation, just watch the miracles flow back to you.

You might be reading this and wanting to give it a go, but still not quite sure. That's okay. First off, focus on your health and fitness. Let's get you feeling better about yourself.

Then when you feel good, we can move onto gratitude, because we all have something to be grateful for. Start with a daily gratitude list and think of three things that you're grateful for every morning. Keep doing that and see how it makes you feel.

Show appreciation. Reframe your thinking. That unexpected bill in the post? Be grateful for the service provided to you.

Once you've got into the habit of gratitude, then you can start to visualise. Remember, it can't do you any harm so you may as well try it! In fact, you have nothing to lose by attempting to change your thoughts.

You can start by visualising smaller positive things before moving on to the bigger stuff. Have fun with it!

Just like with health and fitness, it takes daily practice and repetition.

Try to let go of any skepticism. Let your imagination flow.

Dare to dream.

CHAPTER SIXTEEN

Your kids are watching you!

I WANT TO FINISH THIS BOOK by rounding it off with the most important lesson for me: Your kids are always watching you.

Hopefully, I have equipped you with enough information so that you can go away and speed up, rather than slow down. This will only have a positive effect on your children.

Most of you guys reading this probably have children. I want you to listen carefully when I tell you: they are <u>always</u> observing and copying you.

Remember how we discussed the importance of environment? How we are a product of our surroundings?

Well, this starts at home.

If your kid is lazy, don't be mad if you're the one sat on your arse being a couch potato!

Of course, that may hurt to hear, but this book might be the kick up the bum you need!

You can't blame your kids for being lazy. If you're lazy yourself, you're not encouraging them to exercise.

I'll be honest, I'm a pretty soft dad and I'm always having a laugh with my boys. However, when it comes to activity, it's the only area I am strict – simply because I know how important it is, physically and mentally.

During the lockdown, I've got to admit, our routine with home schooling was terrible. We tried, but it was a bloody challenge, as I'm sure it was for everyone!

I didn't enjoy it because I'm not a school teacher. I didn't like having to put that kind of pressure on my lads. There were loads of times we would sack off the schoolwork and head outside to be active instead.

I'm very, very strong in my message. Even though they're seven and eight, they know about the importance of health and fitness. To stay fit and healthy is to live a happy life.

It's quite challenging to convince two kids to get outside and get active. How can I preach about how it's "good for their mental health to get outside", when they're quite comfortable indoors? They have a loving home environment.

They're close in age and have each other for company. There are many times they'd prefer to be indoors in the warmth, playing their PS4.

However, I simply cannot rest easy in my bed, knowing my kids aren't getting outdoors and being active.

In this day and age, with phones and I-pads, it has never been easier to be a lazy parent. I'm sure there are plenty of times we've let them play on their PS4 all day for a bit of peace!

However, you have to lead. Even if you don't want to, you have to.

My boys have certainly given me plenty of resistance to getting outside. However, when they do get out and hit the fresh air, within ten minutes, the I-pads are forgotten.

I have no doubt that the activity my parents engaged me in at a young age has played a massive part in my life. At around the age of eight or nine, I would go with my mum (two or three times a week) to the aerobics class that she taught. She taught up to thirty or forty ladies at a time. I'd either watch or join in at the back of the class!

That had an effect on me, one hundred per cent. I've no doubt that it gave me the drive to do what I do now at boot camps.

Although I didn't live with my dad for large parts of my childhood, I would see him most weekends. We would always be kicking a football around at the park. He also got involved in helping out with my football training; something I do today with my kids.

Just as kids pick up the positives, they also pick up the negatives.

Remember how I told you about my son (when he was two or three years old) copying me? Remember how I used to get multiple packets of crisps and eat them back-to-back?

That was a dark moment of realization when I knew I had to change and get help. I didn't want those bad habits for my son!

On the contrary, one of the happiest moments was watching my youngest son Elliot compete in a Lidl Mudder event. He was only five years old!

My friend Andy and I had taken the kids to Gloucestershire the day after running in Tough Mudder. We wanted to get our boys involved in the kids' event. The course was extremely muddy and the kids were plastered head to toe in mud!

He was the smallest and youngest of the group and I was anxious he wasn't going to enjoy it. Well, both him and his mate got stuck in and absolutely loved it!

I was brimming with tears of joy and pride as I watched him tackle each obstacle with such determination, carefree to how muddy he was getting!

Again, this isn't to impress you – rather to impress upon you – that he would have seen me coming back from Tough Mudder events over the years covered in mud. A far cry from eating packets of crisps one after the other!

I was always talking to them about such events and showing them videos from an early age. Clearly, it had sunk in!

There were also all those play centers with ropes, obstacles and slides. Places that they wanted me to play with them. It might not have seemed worth it at the time, but in hindsight it clearly was!

For me, the greatest gift in the world, is to be active with my kids. Hands down, it's what I live for. It's the reason I try to stay healthy.

During the first big lockdown, I helped my boys learn how to ride a bike. Then I watched them progress to scooters and skate parks! I took my eldest out on his bike whilst I ran alongside, sometimes for up to 18km. The feeling was incredible.

We'd pack a little bag with energy drinks, chocolate and sweets. We'd make it a fun day, having a pit stop every 2 or 3k, so that he could have another bite of a Yorkie or some jelly babies!

It was the ultimate feeling and really lifted me from the frustration of trying to home-school.

Those memories will always live on and there are many more to make.

I want you to sit for a minute and think about the life you could create with your kids if you got more active with them?

You are going to have to be that example.

Do you want your kids to get off their phones and move more? You are going to have to show them!

Do you want your kids to eat less junk? You're going to have to eat less junk!

You've got to show them!

Children are just waiting to be guided by you and you can begin influencing them now in a positive way!

Show them the way!

It doesn't have to be difficult. I have already told you that simply upping your steps is great for weight loss and overall health.

Walk them to school, walk them back from school just be active with them and see where it takes you!

What if you just started to take your kids to the park? When you get there, don't sit down! Stay active and get involved with them.

They will love you for it!

Printed in Great Britain
by Amazon